Maximum Energy is ab
about life, health probler
you can solve the prol
colossal bonus. Good an

Au

Ted Broer's passion and
informed, down-to-eart
With his dynamic, upbe
promises to make crusad

This is a great book. I
and lifestyle— and I fo
energy, fast, this is the so

MAXIMUM ENERGY

TED BROER

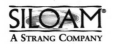

SILOAM
A STRANG COMPANY

MAXIMUM ENERGY by Ted Broer
Published by Siloam
A Strang Company
600 Rinehart Road
Lake Mary, Florida 32746
www.siloam.com

Unless otherwise noted, all Scripture quotations are from the Holy Bible, New Living Translation, copyright © 1996. Used by permission of Tyndale House Publishers, Inc., Wheaton, IL 60189. All rights reserved.

Scripture quotations marked KJV are from the King James Version of the Bible.

Scripture quotations marked NAS are from the New American Standard Bible. Copyright © 1960, 1962, 1963, 1968, 1971, 1972, 1973, 1975, 1977 by the Lockman Foundation. Used by permission.

Library of Congress Catalog Card Number: 99-74173
International Standard Book Number: 0-88419-643-7

This book is not intended to take the place of medical advice and treatment from your personal physician. Readers are advised to consult their own doctor or other qualified health professional regarding the treatment of their medical problems. Neither the publisher nor the author takes any responsibility for any possible consequences from any treatment, action or application of medicine supplement, herb or preparation to any person reading or following the information in this book.

03 04 05 06 07—11 10 9 8 7
Printed in the United States of America

ACKNOWLEDGMENTS

THROUGHOUT OUR LIVES we are faced with decisions that ultimately determine the course and direction of our lives. Upon occasion we all face what I call "crossroads." These are the decisions that have a high impact on the outcome of our lives. Many times these crossroads are difficult to spot when the decision has to be made. In some cases it is only after years of retrospection that we see those crossroads and how our corresponding decisions have had such a dramatic influence on our lives. By these decisions, the tapestry of life is made. Whether this tapestry is one of health and vitality or one of sickness and disease, basically it comes down to the sum total of the decisions we have made.

As I look back at times in my life, there have been several crossroad decisions that have greatly influenced who I am, what I believe and how I live.

The greatest of these took place in 1979 when I became a Christian. It was the greatest single crossroad that I ever encountered, and being such it has affected every area of my life in ways that I could never have imagined.

The second crossroad that I would like to share with you occurred in 1981. This is when I was first privileged to hear Zig Ziglar on audio cassette tapes. The reason I call this a crossroad decision is because of the tremendous impact this great man has had on my life. He taught me the necessity of goal setting, character building and the importance of a healthy self-image. During the past six years I have been privileged to do approximately one hundred seminars with him. I'm here to tell you that he walks his talk, and it has been a honor to know him on both a personal and professional basis.

My third and final crossroad I would like to share with you is when I married my beautiful and wonderful wife, Sharon, in 1984. She has provided so much to my life and has always believed in the endeavors I have chosen to pursue. I also thank her for being such an incredible mother to our two sons, Austin and Harrison.

The reason I am sharing these personal thoughts is twofold. First, I felt I needed to publicly acknowledge them. The second reason is to let you know that if you read this book and apply what you have learned, it can be a crossroad in your pursuit of health, hopefully taking you from sickness and disease to health and vitality in only a few short weeks.

I hope you enjoy reading this book as much as I have enjoyed writing it. Remember, your health is not a destination, but a lifetime journey of crossroads. Make sure you choose well. Your health and the health of your family depend on it.

CONTENTS

PREFACE

THE CONCEPTS IN this book are the product of
my life. They represent the fruit of nearly two
decades of professional research, of experience
working with thousands of clients on a one-to-one
basis and of my personal experience as a twenty-
seven-year-old victim of heart disease—trying to
determine why my life had almost been cut short.

I have devoted my professional life to removing
the confusion and complexity that surround the
subjects of health, nutrition, exercise and physical
energy. Equipped with an extensive education in
the fields of biological science, chemistry, psychology and exercise physiology, as well as extensive
post graduate studies in nutrition and the biochemical makeup of food and how it interacts with our
bodies, I have made every effort to tap the cumulative knowledge and insights of other researchers

and top leaders in these fields. You will notice that in each chapter of this book, the most important principles appear to be very simple. This is no accident. I have had to dig these truths out from under mountains of myth, misinformation and outright deception permeating our culture.

I am convinced that the dynamic health keys in this book will give you a *strategic energy advantage.* They will make a clear and unmistakable difference in your vitality and quality of life, and they will arm you with knowledge so you can make informed choices about what to eat and what not to eat. My goal is to help you develop a lifestyle that promotes and provides maximum energy levels and good health over the long term.

You should know why certain foods or practices may harm your health, rob you of energy, or weaken your immune system. You need to understand why a diet rich in certain high-fat foods can cause heart disease, high blood pressure, cancer, diabetes and countless other health problems. My goal isn't to "take away the things you like" in the name of healthier living. I want to show you the important choices and attractive alternatives available to you so you can live a healthy, energy-filled life that brings you joy and deep satisfaction in all areas of your life—mental, physical and spiritual.

—TED BROER

AUBURNDALE, FLORIDA

Part I:
Vital Keys to
Maximizing Your Energy

SOME OF US HAVE
TO NEARLY LOSE
SOMETHING BEFORE
WE LEARN HOW TO
TREASURE IT.

One

DISCOVERING THE KEYS
TO GOOD HEALTH

I N THE FALL of 1983, I was driving my new Grand
Prix east on Interstate 10, heading for Orlando,
Florida. Everything seemed to be going my way, and
the future looked bright. Suddenly I felt a searing
pain in my chest that surged down my left arm. By
the time I had careened to the side of the road in my
car, my left arm was almost totally numb with pain.

I thought, *Lord, this can't be happening to me! I
am only twenty-seven years old, but I feel like I am
having a heart attack. What is going on? Why is this
happening?*

As I lay helplessly sprawled across the bucket
seats of the Grand Prix, my mind began to register
random impressions and thoughts: This center
floor console is unbelievably hard. . . . It is really
uncomfortable crunched over like this. . . . This is
unbelievable. . . . What am I going to do?

1

I knew I was in serious trouble. There was no way for me to contact anybody (car phones were uncommon in those days, and I didn't have a CB radio). I needed an ambulance and immediate medical care, but I didn't know what to do.

I lay there for about fifteen minutes—it seemed like an eternity.

Finally the pain subsided enough for me to get the car rolling again. When I reached my physician, he immediately ordered an ECG (a test used to measure electrical activity in the heart). When the test results were returned, I was shocked to discover that I was suffering from a disease called *pericarditis,* an inflammation of the pericardial sac that surrounds the heart.

CONFINED TO BED FOR THREE MONTHS

THE DOCTOR TOLD me that my heart had actually become inflamed by a strain of bacteria in my bloodstream. This bacterial infection was deteriorating part of the vital pericardial lining around my heart. This condition was extremely painful, and I really felt that if it were to continue, my life would soon be over.

The doctors gave me prescriptions for several different types of anti-inflammatory drugs and painkillers, but the drugs did absolutely nothing for me. The treatment was not effective, and essentially I remained confined to my bed for almost three months.

You might be thinking, *Well Ted, you must have had some really serious health problems or some very poor health habits to have this happen to you at the age of twenty-seven.* The opposite was true. I had been a competitive athlete all the way through high school and college.

Like most heart disease victims under the age of forty, I could not believe that I had been struck with pericarditis. After all, I had followed a rigorous athletic training program and was seriously committed to maintaining my physical fitness. My primary health habits were excellent—with just a few weak points. (God told Hosea, "My people [perish] for lack of knowledge" [Hos. 4:6, NAS]. I didn't have the knowledge I needed in just a few areas—and I was being destroyed.)

Still, I went from bad to worse during the three months I spent in bed. I gained more than twenty pounds of excess fluid, and my body weight ballooned to over two hundred pounds. I was drinking two bottles of cough syrup daily. My whole body was swollen, including my waistline and face. I felt bad all the time, and I simply did not know what to do. The only thing keeping me going was the eighteen cups of coffee I was drinking daily (more on that later)!

YOU CAN CHANGE THE STATE OF YOUR HEALTH

PERHAPS YOU HAVE experienced the same problems or have faced other health problems that really burdened your body and spirit. There is a simple answer for you in most cases. I have discovered what I did not know when I was twenty-seven years old: Many times we can change the state of our health by simply changing what we put into our system. I am telling you my story in detail because I want you to learn how to make correct choices to avoid the pain associated with a situation similar to mine. Remember that it is always better to walk in divine health than to experience healing.

My life changed the day I received a visit from a friend named Jeff who lived in Daytona Beach. He had asked me to get tickets to the nationally televised NCAA national football championship game between Florida State and Miami (FSU fans will remember that 1983 was the year Miami defeated FSU for the national championship). Jeff had asked if he could stay at my home, and I said, "Sure."

When he arrived at my home he couldn't believe how I had changed. "Ted, what in the world has happened to you?" he said. "You look absolutely terrible. Look at you...you are swollen and puffy, and you can't stop coughing."

"Jeff, I am in really bad shape, and I just don't know what to do about it," I said. "I have to take an incredible amount of Sudafed just to breathe, and I put down bottles of cough syrup every single day." On top of that, every day I was taking painkillers and anti-inflammatory medicine prescribed by my doctors. Yet despite all the medication and bed rest, I was growing progressively worse.

Since Jeff was my guest for the game that weekend, I ordered pizza for everyone that night. It was covered with my favorite topping, pepperoni. I was surprised to see Jeff picking off all the pepperoni slices, but I just added them to my pizza so they wouldn't "go to waste."

Jeff was a nutritionist, and after he had listened to my story about how my health had deteriorated, he started talking about health and nutrition. He knew I had been in the health field for many years and that I thought I knew quite a bit about health at that time. I had been a competitive bodybuilder, and I had just completed work on degrees in biology, chemistry and exercise physiology as well as an MBA from Florida State University.

Maybe that explains why Jeff was so blunt and direct when he told me, "Ted, the problem with you is that you are eating the wrong types of foods. You are eating too many unclean meats, and I've also noticed that you are drinking about eighteen cups of coffee a day."

I shook my head and said, "Jeff, I know you are really health- and nutrition-conscious, and I understand that you have helped a lot of people, but I don't think this is a dietary problem. In fact, I talked to the doctors, and they told me that my heart was the problem." Jeff didn't seem to be impressed, so I added, "They assured me that my problem has nothing to do with my diet. They also said there was nothing that I could do except take the anti-inflammatory drugs and the medicines they prescribed."

Jeff looked closely at my swollen face and bloated body, and then he said, "Ted, let me ask you a question: *Is what you are doing working?*"

All I could say was, "Well, obviously not. I am growing progressively sicker, and I don't know what to do. In fact, I really feel that if something doesn't change, then I am going to die. Frankly, I don't know if I am going to see my twenty-eighth birthday."

HIGH LEVELS OF TOXINS

JEFF SMILED AND said, "Ted, I found some really interesting research years ago when I first started working. These research studies talked about pork, high-fat luncheon meat, shellfish and a lot of other problem foods in the diet."

I was thinking, *Oh, no. Is he starting on my pork and shellfish? I love pork chops, and I love shellfish.*

Then suddenly I remembered that after eating at a golf country club two years earlier in Haines City, Florida, I had become deathly ill for five days with shellfish poisoning.

Jeff continued, describing the very high levels of toxins, cholesterol and fat contained in pork and shellfish. He said that the human body really wasn't made to assimilate these kinds of foods. Naturally, I had to ask, "Now, Jeff, can you *document* your claim that these things weren't made for the body to assimilate?"

Jeff knew I was a Christian, so he started off with a heavyweight source. "Ted, did you know that even God told us in the Bible that we shouldn't eat certain types of food?"

I quickly pulled out the usual pat answer for this kind of statement, saying, "Look, Jeff, that has nothing to do with us today. Those guidelines are thousands of years old. We don't have to live by those dietary laws any longer."

"I used to think the same thing, Ted. But then I started doing a lot of research," Jeff said. "I found out that the foods the Bible tells us not to eat are still not very healthy for us today."

Sick as I was, I was still too stubborn to go down without a fight. "What kind of research did you do?" I asked.

Jeff responded that he had a clinic in Daytona Beach and had worked with hundreds of patients.

He had found immune system diseases in many of his patients who consumed unclean meats and shellfish.

"I Don't Know If I Buy All This Stuff"

"Well, that is interesting," I said, "but I don't know if I buy all this stuff."

Jeff just shrugged and said, "Well, Ted, that is up to you. I am just telling you what I have learned over the past few years. If you will avoid the unclean meats, drink distilled water, cut out the coffee and decrease your stress, then I believe you will see these physical symptoms clear up quickly. If you want to apply this and see if it will help you, then go ahead. If you don't want to, then don't."

Jeff left, and I started looking at my lifestyle. I looked at my diet, and from a biblical perspective I didn't like what I saw. Frankly, I've never responded well to negative arguments about high-fat foods or the dangers of "burning the candle at both ends" in a fast-paced lifestyle. But this time, I wanted something *positive*—I wanted my life back. I wanted my energy and health back. I wanted to look good and feel good again! (I wouldn't be surprised if you feel the same way.)

Armed with a driving motivation to regain my health and energy along with a reasonable hope for a long life, I examined my lifestyle with honesty.

The first thing I noticed was that I was drinking a lot of coffee. I was drinking up to eighteen cups of coffee a day. That is a *lot* of coffee. (I didn't realize that according to the English medical journal *Lancet* just five cups of coffee a day in a man could increase his risk of heart disease by up to 50 percent.)

I was using the caffeine that occurs naturally in coffee as a stimulant in my body. My goal was to increase my energy, and I methodically overdosed my system with large amounts of coffee to reach that goal. At the time, I didn't realize that the caffeine could overload my adrenal system. In fact, according to Mary Lou Retton, Carl Lewis and Bonnie Blair—all Olympic gold medal winners with whom I regularly conduct seminars—caffeine is a banned substance in Olympic competition.

I began to realize that some of the basic principles of nutritional health had somehow escaped me. *Maybe Jeff was right,* I thought to myself. *Maybe I've been eating the wrong types of food and abusing my body. Maybe I do need to change my lifestyle.* Obviously, what I was doing wasn't working.

Even at that early stage, I knew better than to "change just my *diet.*" The first three letters of diet are "d-i-e." I still don't endorse diets today. I endorse a healthy lifestyle, which includes healthy living and healthy eating habits that allow us to feel good every single day and to live a life filled with vibrant energy.

I decided to give Jeff's ideas a try. I couldn't get his final question out of my head: *"Let me ask you this, Ted: Are the things you are doing now working?"*

A STRING OF SMALL CHOICES

LIFE CONSISTS OF a series of choices. The little choices that we make on a day-to-day basis are the same factors that affect our health tomorrow, next year or in the next decade. Someone attending one of my health seminars once asked me, "How important is it to watch your diet all the time?"

"Look," I said. "It is not what you eat from Christmas to New Year's that determines your health—even though it may affect it a little bit. It is what you eat from New Year's to Christmas that matters the most."

In other words, the long-term picture of your health is created by all the things that you do and don't do and all the things that you put and don't put into your body on a day-to-day basis. This ongoing string of small choices can determine whether you are going to be healthy or sick in the days ahead. Genetic factors influence the equation in some ways, but the health and nutrition choices you make today can still help determine whether you end up battling heart disease, diabetes or cancer tomorrow. How can I make such a claim? Study after study has shown clearly that cancer, diabetes, heart disease and hypertension, in most cases, *are related either directly or indirectly to nutrition.* If these diseases are *caused* in part or in whole by our nutritional choices, then doesn't it make sense that they can be *prevented* in part or in whole by better choices?

Whether we like it or not, you and I have important choices to make every time we sit down at the dinner table or evaluate our physical appearance in a mirror. In this book, I am determined to give you information you need to make *informed* choices about your health and lifestyle.

Robbed of my health and energy at the age of twenty-seven, I was desperate to find a solution. Without energy, it is difficult to live a fulfilling life. I began an aggressive program to adopt the new food and lifestyle choices Jeff had recommended. It took me a year to regain my energy fully, but the benefits of my lifestyle change started appearing almost immediately. In less than a month I experienced obvious improvement in the way I felt and looked! It was during this time that I knew I had found my mission in life—I just had to try to help people avoid the mess in which I had landed. I wanted to help bring relief and hope to people who were already battling life-threatening health problems linked to both nutritional and physiological problems.

God's Wisdom Is Confirmed by Science

AFTER CENTURIES OF scientific research, so-called "modern man" is coming full circle to acknowledge the eternal truths in God's Word concerning physics, marriage, finances, relationships, prosperity, morality, history and nutrition. Such conservative organizations as the American Heart Association, the American Cancer Society and the American Diabetes Association have spent billions of dollars on research in the last few decades. Researchers have finally recognized that excessive dietary saturated fat levels and poor nutrition contribute directly to the development and advancement of cardiovascular disease, cancer and diabetes. It is clear that the heart of our health problem has to do with our approach to health. It is time for us—patients and healthcare professionals alike—to shift our emphasis from the *treatment* of disease to the *prevention* of disease.

It is clear that our Western diet has some serious problems associated with it. Every year, national organizations and government agencies issue dietary guidelines that seem to grow closer and closer to the dietary guidelines God gave to Moses in the Old Testament thousands of years ago. It is no accident that God's wisdom is being "confirmed" by the latest scientific findings.

Most of us realize we need to make wise lifestyle

decisions based on a long-term viewpoint, but most Americans are uneducated or misinformed about nutrition and diet—along with the American media in general. I suspect that many of our medical doctors are confused about nutrition, but many would never admit it openly.

At every turn we are bombarded with conflicting nutritional information. One government study is released, telling us one thing, and a week later another study from a different source releases, telling us the exact opposite. Which do you believe?

Let me give you an example. For fifteen years I have warned people who attend our seminars, listen to my national radio broadcasts or watch my prime-time television shows that partially hydrogenated oils such as those contained in margarine, shortening and peanut butter are absolutely terrible for their health.

Then over the years "new studies" hit the news services, and news commentators around the country told millions of viewers that butter had been proven to be bad for the human body. What was their solution? They told health-conscious viewers that margarine was the best way to go. (No one seemed to think it was important to tell us that the new study had been funded and conducted by the nation's margarine manufacturers.) Remember, margarine was originally developed during the war years when there was a scarcity of butter. Margarine that looks like Crisco would be sent to homes with a tube of yellow dye included to make it look like butter. Again, the government unknowingly included a product that could later help us to lead the world when it comes to heart disease and cancer.

Finally, after all these years of warning the American population about partially hydrogenated oils and trans fats, the Harvard School of Public Health has come out on my side stating that an additional thirty thousand people die in the U.S. each year from heart disease because of their consumption.

DOES IT LINE UP TO *THE TRUTH?*

WHENEVER YOU HEAR something new about nutrition or harmful substances, it is critical to *consider the source.* Look for multiple witnesses who support the same conclusion. Be aware that every study rises or falls by its impartial methodology. This last criterion is almost impossible to monitor, but without it, the research is probably worthless.

In every area of life, including the areas of nutrition, food and lifestyle choices and human relationships, my first accountability is to the Word of God. Everything and everybody else need to line up behind that rock-solid source of truth.

However, even though we have been warned for many years about the importance of nutrition, many of us simply never listened. Let me give you an example as far back as 1976, when the U.S. Department of Agriculture (USDA) issued a report from Dr. Mark Hecksted of the Harvard School of Public Health that contained this comment:

> I wish to stress that there is a great deal of evidence that continues to accumulate, which strongly implicates, and in some instances proves, that the major causes of death and disability in the United States are related to the diet that we eat. I include coronary artery disease, heart disease (which accounts for nearly half of the deaths in the United States), several of the most important forms of cancer, hypertension, diabetes and obesity, as well as other chronic diseases.[1]

If you have never heard this statement quoted before, I am not surprised. I didn't hear about it until 1983 when I read it in *The McDougall Plan*, a book by Dr. John A. McDougall and his wife, Mary. I wanted to know *why* I had never heard this statement or anything like it in the national media or in my professional studies. Dr. Hecksted's statement was quoted in an official government publication listing the "Dietary Goals for the United States"!

I discovered that the various food lobbies in the United States know that many of the products they sell to Americans are not healthy; however, they don't want their profits endangered by comments like the one made by Dr. Hecksted. The overriding issue for them doesn't appear to be truth or ethical conduct—it is profit.

THE TRUTH WAS SUPPRESSED

JOHN MCDOUGALL IS a medical doctor, a board-certified internist and medical examiner who served as assistant clinical professor at the University of Hawaii School of Medicine. In his landmark book, *The McDougall Plan,* he made a surprising observation and revelation that really challenged me to find the truth beyond the hype:

> Large industries have great influence in high places. They are government subsidized when their profits go below a certain point, even if the reason for failure is that people won't buy their products because of health hazards.
>
> The dairy and meat industries are presently suffering from a depressed market as a direct result of increased public awareness. Officials of the U.S. government... actually have suppressed printed material intended to improve health because of the

material's potential harmfulness to business. Food lobbyists had little trouble convincing the Department of Agriculture to abandon publication of a relatively noncontroversial pamphlet, *Food/2,* which recommended ways to reduce fat and cholesterol in the American diet by discouraging meat, poultry, dairy, egg, fat and oil consumption.[2]

Why did these lobbyists feel it was important to ban this publication? Obviously they feared it would affect the bottom line—the sales and profits—of their corporate clients. They believed that if it affected the bottom line, it would also affect the stockholders, corporate shareholders and everyone else who wanted to see higher sales and income. Ultimately a sales slump affects jobs, so the lobbyists were able to sway the Department of Agriculture enough to get this scientifically based food pamphlet pulled off the government printing presses.

Frankly, this kind of back room wheeling and dealing nauseates me. This pamphlet, *Food/2,* was designed to tell the American people the truth about nutrition, and the truth is what set me free when I learned about health and nutrition from Jeff.

I don't want you or anyone else to go through what I did. You shouldn't have to reach the verge of death to discover the simple truth about good health. We can enjoy maximum energy and optimum health throughout our lives, and the keys to this kind of life are very simple. As with most things worthwhile, the way to get maximum energy is to do it one choice at a time.

I would now like to ask you a simple question that I ask the hundreds of thousands who attend my seminars and the millions who listen to my radio and television broadcasts each year: If you are twenty, thirty or even one hundred pounds over-weight, or if you just feel terrible with no energy or zest for life, and if you continue doing what you have done to get where you are, why do you think your results are going to be different? If you are going east on the interstate, but you want to go west, you're not going to get to where you want to go unless you turn around. If you step off a ten-story building, you will always go down. It doesn't matter whether you believe in the law of gravity or not. So please continue to read this book with an open mind; let's make the correct choices for your health one decision at a time.

MOST OF THE FOOD IN AMERICA TODAY WILL SUPPORT LIFE, BUT IT WON'T SUSTAIN HEALTH. [1]

Two

SUPPORT LIFE
OR SUSTAIN HEALTH?

THE HUMAN BODY is a masterpiece, a biological and chemical wonder that still baffles and awes the scientific and medical communities of the world. The majority of our most accomplished physicians and surgeons are quick to admit that they do not really understand how the body functions or heals itself in times of stress or trauma—but they know it does.

From its moment of conception to its final moments of life, the human body demands energy to function. This superb biochemical machine is part of the Creator's master design. How much energy do our bodies need, and where does the energy come from? Let me begin with this very simple equation: When you supply your body with *maximum energy,* you get *maximum output.* The formula is "energy in vs. energy out." In this area, we all want to have a "positive" equation.

Our bodies live and die at the cellular level. It is a fundamental principle that your body contains from forty to seventy trillion cells. They are all interrelated and work together like a large, semi-permeable, porous membrane integrated into a bioelectrical field. Your body is so intricately "wired" that if you rub a fresh clove of garlic on the bottom of your foot, within twenty minutes you will literally *taste* the garlic in your mouth! In the same way, when a person with a heart condition feels his or her heart begin to beat irregularly, if he or she slips a nitroglycerin tablet under the tongue, within seconds that drug will be transported directly from the mouth to the heart, helping to regulate the rhythm of that fluctuating heartbeat!

Each body cell requires oxygen, nutrients, minerals and several different types of amino acids to function properly (and these are only a few of the requirements). When these key components are missing from or deficient in your system for any reason, as a whole your body will become progressively weaker and can eventually die. Your cells also produce and interact with many other components such as hormones, enzymes, urea and carbon dioxide. Some of these things are toxins that are eliminated constantly from the body under normal conditions in order to maintain proper health.

Problems arise when your body cells become over-loaded with so many toxins that they cannot be eliminated from the system, or when insufficient oxygen reaches the cells for some reason.

Some of the key advances in our understanding of the human cell have demonstrated that human body cells become weak and may die or mutate when they are denied adequate oxygen.

Researchers have theorized that the cell could possibly live forever if toxins could be kept away from the cell while all the necessary nutrients were provided on an ongoing basis. In my opinion, this theory is supported by the Creation account in the Book of Genesis. I believe God designed Adam's body (and therefore its cells) to last forever. God's original intent was for Adam (and his offspring) to live forever, and it is reasonable to conclude that the Master Designer also created Adam's body as a vehicle or physical dwelling with eternal existence and service in mind.

When Adam and Eve fell from a sinless condition in the Garden of Eden, the consequence was that the grim reality of death and cell degeneration and toxemia entered the human equation. From that point on, we see the human life span shrinking steadily and the appearance of untimely and sorrowful death caused by violence, human excess, ravaging human diseases and the sheer difficulty of survival in a fallen world.

Dr. Alexis Carrel, a Nobel Prize-winning medical doctor and researcher, devised a unique experiment involving a cluster of chicken embryo heart cells. By ensuring that the cell cluster received enough oxygen and that metabolic waste products were removed on a regular basis, he was able to keep the cells alive for *over twenty years* in a laboratory petri dish! These cells continued to live until the day one of the research assistants forgot to remove the cellular waste. That was the day the chicken heart cells suddenly died in their own waste products.[2]

At the very least, this experiment illustrates why it is so important for the human body to eliminate cellular toxins on a regular basis. (The human body normally accomplishes this through proper lung aeration achieved through consistent exercise, proper colon function marked by regular large bowel movements every day and proper kidney function.) Dr. Carrel may have been one of the greatest minds of our century, and I believe that within the next few years his basic cellular theories will be shown to have been accurate to even our most skeptical scientists.

Remember, the body eliminates toxins in four basic ways: through the skin, the lungs, the kidneys and the colon. What does this have to do with energy levels in the body? If our bodies are toxic, we can experience all types of side effects ranging from lethargy to headaches. We must make sure that the temple God has given us stays pure in order to maximize our energy and our health.

Many people do not realize that *it requires energy to digest the food we eat.* In fact, the digestive process is one of the primary energy drains on the body! This is why our food choices play such a major role in determining our energy levels and state of health.

Let me give you a simple example to show you how this works. If you eat a carrot, your digestive system will require a certain amount of energy to properly digest that carrot (which includes withdrawing its nutrients, absorbing the water in it and disposing of the remainder). The upside of this energy withdrawal is that the nutrients extracted from that carrot will also give your body a certain amount of energy after it is digested. If the carrot has the potential to give you ten units of energy (I've selected this even number at random for illustration purposes), and it takes two units of energy for your body to digest the carrot, then you would have a net increase of eight units of energy after you have digested the carrot.

The American diet primarily consists of rich foods. By rich foods, I am referring to foods that contain heavy concentrations of fat, protein, carbohydrates (especially sugar) and sodium. This includes foods such as marbled red meat, poultry, pork, eggs, high-fat dairy products, processed foods containing highly refined flours and shellfish. Research has shown that many of these rich foods require tremendous amounts of energy for our bodies to digest and eliminate their cellular residues. It is ironic that these rich foods were once reserved for special holidays or occasions of celebration, while the bulk of the American diet used to consist of basic whole-grain foods, vegetables and less-expensive (and lower-fat) meats accompanied by water. Affluent societies in the United States and abroad have reversed this picture with rich foods becoming our everyday fare. The change has been costly.

As you will see later in this book, I am not against eating red meat, but I do advise you to wisely limit the amount and frequency of red meat in your diet. Why? One reason has to do with this relationship between energy gained and energy expended. If you decide to eat a large portion of red meat just before you go to bed tonight—which is the worst time to eat anything—your body must exert a certain amount of energy to digest that meat. Red meat is difficult to digest and contains far more protein and fat than your body actually needs (I'll explain why I say this a little later in the book), so let's say your digestive system can potentially retrieve fifty units of energy from that steak.

It sounds like a lot of energy when you think about it, but have you ever heard people make the following comment? "You know, whenever I eat a heavy meal with steak or roast, it just seems to stay with me. I don't seem to get hungry afterward." That statement is very accurate, and this is why: The human body has to struggle to digest red meat. That large juicy steak can give you fifty units of energy (yes, I am quick to acknowledge that steak can taste *very* good at times), but it will take a large percentage of the energy and a very long time for your digestive system to digest it and then eliminate it. After all that time and energy expenditure, depending on your digestive system, you may only retrieve a minimum increase in energy!

If you consider how hard your body has worked—and worked and worked some more throughout the night while you tossed and turned—you will realize that many meals are an insignificant source of energy. You may be surprised to know that your body was designed to run primarily on *complex carbohydrates*—of which steak contains zero. The carbohydrate food groups include grains (and grain products such as whole-grain breads, pasta and cereals), fruit, vegetables, beans, legumes and potatoes.

If we are serious about increasing our energy levels, that means you and I need to reduce (notice that I did not say *eliminate*) the amount of animal protein in our diets. You might as well know right now that I am not a vegetarian. I still eat animal proteins, but since I demand maximum energy from my body and have an active lifestyle, I have shifted my focus away from inefficient energy sources in favor of high-energy foods such as the complex carbohydrates group.

When I say that the human body was designed to run primarily on carbohydrates, I am not including refined, processed carbohydrates like Hostess Twinkies, snack cakes or cupcakes. (I will discuss these foods in detail later on, but let me say that these foods have very little if any nutritive value and should be avoided.)

If we want to have more energy for our bodies each day and do not have a weight problem, we need to increase our intake of high-energy complex carbohydrates such as fresh fruits, vegetables, whole grains and legumes. These high-fiber foods help the body function at peak efficiency, and they provide the human body with tremendous amounts of potential energy and protective vitamins in return.

Body Cell Life

As we learned earlier, everything in the physical body begins and ends at the cellular level. For this reason, we need to understand that there are several different ways our body cells can die.

Oxygen loss

First, body cells can quickly die when they are deprived of oxygen for even a short period. Wherever I go, people constantly ask me, "What is the most important thing that we do as living beings?"

They are almost always surprised when I say, "Breathe." I say this because oxygen is the most vital component necessary to sustain life in a human cell. Under most circumstances, a human being deprived of oxygen will die within a matter of minutes.

Water loss

On the other hand, the average healthy person can go without water for a day or so before serious or fatal damage is done to the cells of major body organs. For this reason, water is the second most vital substance for the cell.

Nutrient loss

Most people in good health can go without food or nutrients for several weeks and still survive.[3] This explains why food and nutrients are ranked third in order of the cell's dependence scale.

Electrical disturbance

Body cells will also die if their electrical field is disturbed. Many people are surprised to learn that

29

human cells, and the human body as a whole, contain electrical charges. The human body actually resonates a very specific and measurable electrical field and electronic frequency. The electrical field of an individual cell can be disturbed through a potassium or sodium imbalance, or when the body sustains an electrical shock. These disturbances can bring rapid or instant death to the cell.

Rupture

The fifth way by which a cell can die is by rupture. This happens every day when children fall down and scrape their knees or fall off a bicycle. It happens to adults when they bump a shin against some furniture. Major cell trauma occurs when a human body suffers a gunshot wound, which ruptures millions of body cells, often with fatal results. Cells are also ruptured by invasive virus cells that are equipped with sharp whiplike appendages designed to puncture the wall of a target host cell. Under normal circumstances, the body's normal defense and maintenance systems efficiently dispose of damaged or dead cells (and invading viruses), and healthy cells quickly multiply to replace the cells lost.

Body cells can also begin to die through atrophy or lack of use. This is what happens when we have a decreased work load. For this reason I urge people *not* to decrease their work loads when they retire because they may actually experience premature death as a result. Atrophy or lack of motion is an enemy of energy in the human body!

I am convinced that Americans in general have a very misinformed concept of the role of rest and relaxation in the healthy lifestyle. We were never meant to adopt a state of constant physical rest as a lifestyle—it leads to premature death!

How many times have you heard of people who led active, healthy lives... *until they retired.* Then after only two or three years go by, we hear that their health and energy levels literally fell apart, and they died prematurely. (Don't retire too early, but if you do, don't become a couch potato.) Again, remember that a decreased work load for your cellular structure can actually cause your body cells to atrophy and become weaker.

How does all this fit into the larger picture? Far too many of us die prematurely because our bodies are deprived of adequate supplies of oxygen, water, food and nutrients necessary to our diets. Your body uses blood to deliver the essential components of oxygen, water and nutrients to your individual body cells. When the blood supply to your cells is diminished due to the narrowing of your arteries because of a lifelong high-saturated-fat food problem and a lack of regular exercise, then your cellular structure will be diminished as well. Your blood flows through an incredibly complex circulatory system that includes your heart, major arteries, veins and the tiny capillary systems distributed throughout your body.

It is important for you to know that when your blood fails to reach a cell in adequate quantities, then that cell is also receiving inadequate supplies of oxygen, water, essential nutrients, vitamins and minerals. At that point the cell will become weakened and will eventually die.

All the factors we have discussed become even more crucial as we move further along in the natural process of aging, because body toxins from a lack of circulation can more easily accumulate in our bodies as we grow older. We will discuss these things in later chapters, but in general we need to make sure our skin is kept free from grease and other types of oil, which will help to ensure our skin breathes properly. Doing so helps our body to eliminate toxins. We need to make sure we get a lot of good fresh air and natural light on our skin as well. (I'm not telling you to rush outside at midday to get a third-degree sunburn! Get just enough sunshine to make sure your skin and body stay healthy. We were not made to spend our lives hiding in man-made caves.) Finally, you should also make sure that your kidneys are working properly by drinking one-half of your body weight in ounces of reverse-osmosis or distilled drinking water daily.

The human body is equipped with a marvelous defense system that is able to repel or overcome almost every major disease or sickness under normal circumstances. Medical research studies are confirming in increasing numbers and frequency that a healthy diet and regular exercise play a major role in the body's long-term resistance to debilitating disease and sickness.

The medical world is divided according to several different theories about what actually causes sickness and disease. One theory maintains that individual human body cells begin to weaken and die when they lack the key components we have just discussed. This gradually leads to the death of the individual. Another theory, called the "germ theory," says that cells die when a germ (a single- or multiple-cell microorganism) successfully evades the body's defense system and invades body cells. This causes the entire body to become weakened, sometimes with fatal results.

Basically, I have found that germs have a very difficult time attacking a healthy body. A perfect example is when everyone in a family is exposed to a "germ," but not everyone gets sick. Germs do exist, and they obviously play a key role in the genesis and advancement of disease. However, it seems to me that these two theories are compatible, not incompatible. The "health theory" includes the basic tenets of the "germ theory," asserting that germs do exist, but have a difficult time success-fully overcoming a person whose body is healthy and getting all the adequate nutrition and exercise that it needs.

This brings us to the next chapter, where we will discuss what I consider to be the most vital keys for maximizing your energy and maintaining optimum health.

PURE WATER COMES
CLOSER TO BEING
A GENUINE HEALTH
POTION THAN ANY
OTHER SUBSTANCE
ON OUR PLANET.

Three

PURE WATER:
THE GREATEST OF ALL
"HEALTH POTIONS"

DO YOU REMEMBER the stories about adventurers who risked their lives and fortunes searching for the mythical fountain of youth? The men in these stories believed there was a fountain where the water was so pure and magical that it could grant them eternal youth—if they could just find it. I can imagine what the term, "health potion," conjures up in your mind, but believe it or not, pure water comes closer to being a genuine health potion than any other substance on our planet!

There is no magic involved, unless you use the term to describe the advanced technology and effort required to produce absolutely pure water in our polluted world. You have to drink an abundance of pure water if you want to be healthy because dehydration, or the lack of pure water in the body, has been a contributing factor in many diseases.

Water purification has become a major issue with our growing problem of water contamination. Did you know that the world's water supply *today* contains the same amount of water it contained *a million years ago?* The volume doesn't change; it *simply recycles.* Unfortunately, the earth's built-in water purifying system has become clogged and overloaded. We have even created new contaminants and chemical substances that the earth has never before encountered. In spite of the problems we face with our water supplies, it is vital that we find reliable sources of pure water to protect our health.

When you talk to people about unsafe drinking water, many of them think of the Black Death, a plague that swept through much of Europe in the 1500s. It was carried primarily by polluted drinking water in an era when mankind was essentially unaware of the existence of germs. (It was also an era when the immune systems of entire groups were destroyed because their main source of food was lard—pig fat—pie. An interesting side note is that Jews in Europe who did not eat pork fat pie weren't dying from the Black Death. In fact, a great persecution arose against the Jews because the victims of the plague thought the "healthy Jews" had placed a curse on them. Again, God's

Word is always right!) Others may think of remote locations such as Sudan, Rwanda, the Amazonian basin or the interior of Mexico, where modern water-purification systems are nonexistent.

Everyone agrees that we need safe water supplies to live healthy lives, but very few people know the facts about the water supplies in modern, state-of-the-art America. Fred Van Lue, a pure-water advocate and technical specialist in the area of water purification and contamination, has learned that United States water treatment plants that handle water for over 90 percent of America do not have any modern technology to treat the water. The term *modern technology* refers to new developments, techniques or equipment discovered or designed *within the last one hundred years.* That means that nine out of every ten municipal water treatment plants in America are operating the same way with the same basic equipment, chemicals and knowledge that they had one hundred years ago!

That means they are essentially limited to removing only organic waste from the water. Most treatment plants don't have the technology to remove *chemical contaminants* from our tap water. Some of them use alum to remove some of the heavy metals, and that isn't necessarily bad. But they are unable to remove the aluminum—a by-product of alum—that this process adds to the water. So while these water treatment plants have successfully removed some of the heavy metals, they have also raised the amount of aluminum consumed every day by the people in their cities.

It is likely that the increased aluminum is contributing to the growing epidemic of Alzheimer's disease in this country. Studies involving the autopsies of deceased Alzheimer's patients have found that the majority of Alzheimer's victims autopsied had high levels of aluminum in their brain tissues.[1]

This should make residents of larger cities like New York City sleep better. According to Van Lue, many large metropolitan cities are using aluminum silicate to help coat the metal water pipes and pipejoints in their sprawling water supply systems to protect them from acidic surface water used for the public water supply. The aluminum silicate works by putting a protective scale inside those pipes. It also mucks up water filters, which is how Fred Van Lue learned about it.

After his son nearly died from fluoride poisoning, Fred set out to learn everything he could about the chemicals and contaminants in our water systems. He used what he learned to design and manufacture some of the most advanced home-use water purification systems in the world. His customers began calling him when his state-of-the-art filters began getting clogged up because they were filtering out so much aluminum silicate.[2]

Some 63 percent of all water sources contain significant levels of organic, heavy metal and chemical contaminants, including lead and mercury. Even if you live on a farm and are using well water, there is no reason that you should think that you're safe. In fact, some of the most lethal water in America is found in the wells of our rural areas. At least city water supplies tend to meet a minimum standard of purity—just killing you *slowly* by increasing the risk of arterial plaquing and depressing your immune systems.

Well water can contain the nitrates from agricultural fertilizers and pesticides in much higher quantities than city water. Watchdog consumer groups based in Washington, D.C., have shown that this is especially likely in the summer months of the growing season. All of the farm-belt states have a dramatic increase in the levels of chemicals, pesticides and nitrates during the growing season because of the runoff from farm lands.

It may surprise you to learn that golf courses are another major source of contamination for municipal water supplies and wells. When I took up golf as a sport, I fell in love with the relaxation and outdoors environment of the sport, but I was shocked to find that I could literally smell the chemicals that groundskeepers use to keep those greens "green." I personally believe they use more chemical products per acre of soil than any other agricultural or industrial group in the country, although it appears that some of the clubs and courses in the industry are trying to cut back on their chemical use.[3]

Sixty-five percent of your body is composed of water; your muscles are 75 percent water. That is why it is so important for us to drink enough water when we are exercising—weight loss and sufficient water consumption are interrelated and interdependent. We always tell the patients starting our Eat, Drink and Be Healthy Program or the Forever Fit at 20, 30, 40 & Beyond Program that the consumption of water is absolutely critical to success.

I make it a point to give this warning to athletes: "If you get thirsty during a workout or competition, you are already dehydrated—it's already too late! The chances are that you are going to start cramping very soon after that sensation of thirst. The right way to handle water consumption is to sip on pure water continually throughout your workout, track meet, marathon or sporting event."

The same advice applies if you are involved in any form of consistent, long-term athletic event or activity such as snow or water skiing, running, cycling, basketball or tennis. Water keeps you from becoming dehydrated, and it really helps your tissues function at their peak performance. The changes that have been made in nationally televised marathons are noticeable. The conventional wisdom preached to young runners by coaches in past years was, "Don't drink any water; you will get a cramp." Now they have water at every station along the route. Times change with increased knowledge and experience.

There is a good reason to drink water while you train. Your body has to store water when it burns calories. In fact, it has to store *3 to 4 grams of water* with every 1 gram of muscle glycogen stored or burned. If you don't have the water available to store the blood sugar you need during exercise, you will deplete your glycogen stores without replenishing them. If you can't get enough water to the cells, you can't have proper cell respiration.

How Much Water Should I Drink?

I RECOMMEND THAT every day you drink at least half of your body weight in ounces of pure water. If you weigh two hundred pounds, then you need to drink at least 100 ounces of pure water a day. If you weigh one hundred forty pounds, you need to drink a minimum of 70 ounces of pure water each day. (When we go snow skiing, my wife and I bring water with us up on the slopes, and we drink water constantly all day.) If you drink that amount of water, you'll reduce feeling tired or sore the next day, because your muscles are not depleted of glycogen. The same thing is true if you are going to have a really intense workout in the gym. Take some bottled water into the gym with you. *Don't drink the tap water out of the chlorine dispensing machines*—also known as the water fountains there. You don't need to put all that chlorine into your body; chlorine is a poison (we cover this in chapter eighteen).

What Is the Best Source of Pure Water?

Once you've made up your mind to give your body the best water available, you face a bewildering set of choices. Which way should you go: spring water, tap water from the municipal treatment plant, reverse-osmosis water or distilled water? All of them claim to be "pure," including your municipal water authority. Should you buy water at the local grocery store, buy a device to purify water at home or pay a water service to bring it to your home?

People will often tell me, "Well, we have reduced our risk of chlorine exposure by buying bottled spring water." The problem is that the bottled water industry is essentially self-regulated, and the government standards they are asked to meet are pretty lax. On top of that, labeling laws or regulations are very easy to manipulate.

BOTTLERS MAY ADD A LITTLE CHLORINE

IF YOU LOOK closely at many of the labels of water products, underneath the dramatic name with its images of sparkling mountain streams fed by allegedly pure sources, you may find a statement like, "Filtered water from municipal water supply of Anytown, USA" or "Spring water from such-and-such a source." In many cases, water bottlers will add a little chlorine as a sanitizer to help extend the shelf life of the product and to protect against organisms that could start breeding in the water.

Fred Van Lue says that bottled spring water is his last choice for drinking water because it is the least treated of all bottled waters. It still has many of the dissolved solids (generously called minerals that are really dissolved rocks and metals) in the water. They are almost totally indigestible because they are in a positively charged metallic state and are up to two thousand times larger than their plant kingdom counterparts, such as organic calcium or selenium.[4]

Our cells can use any of these minerals when they come from the plant kingdom because they are much smaller and possess a cell-friendly negative charge. Positively charged metallic forms of these minerals from the rock kingdom that are found in water interfere with the body's natural function and must be eliminated by the digestive system.

Since municipally treated water and bottled spring water have been ruled out, we are left with two types of water that are fit for human consumption in the modern era: water that has been purified by reverse osmosis or steam-distilled water. If you buy distilled water from a store, you will inevitably end up getting a plastic taste along with your water. That is because pure water is a universal solvent. When packed in plastic, it will begin absorbing the plastic molecules, giving you all of the benefits of plastic in your distilled water. Try to find a local supplier who delivers steam-distilled water in glass containers.

Or you may want to invest in a reverse-osmosis in-home system for water purification. These units come in many different forms and varieties. (I personally recommend the many varieties manufactured by Fred Van Lue's company.) Some units are made to fit right on the end of your kitchen faucet, which will effectively filter out chlorine and microscopic organic contaminants. Other units are designed to attach to your faucet with a hose and provide sparkling clear, reverse-osmosis water in carafes within an hour or so. Larger under-the-sink units filter much larger amounts of water in "real time" and provide a much wider range of filtering and extraction processes.

WHAT DO YOU DO WHEN YOUR WATER IS BAD?

MY WIFE AND I live in Florida in an area with a very high water table—and very bad water. All our water comes from a ground well, and the scaling was terrible (not to mention the taste). We finally invested in a WaterWise "whole house unit" that provides pure water for our entire house. Not everyone will want or need to make that kind of investment, but in our case, we feel that it is a lifesaver.

Many of the harmful substances in our water supplies are not easy to remove (still another reason why they should never have been *added* in the first place). Fortunately, chlorine is one of the elements that is easy to remove if you have the right system. Let me make it clear that I am *not* talking about a water softener. Water softeners are promoted as the great answer to hard water and scaling, but I call them *glorified consumer toys.* They do not remove all chlorine, and they add very high levels of salt to the water, which may also be absorbed through the skin every time you shower or bathe or even wash your face. The human body treats salt in this form as a toxin, unlike the sodium found naturally in our fruits and vegetables.

While trying to adapt technology for home use, Fred Van Lue also developed the electrostatic precipitator to prevent scaling. His goal at the time was to eliminate the use of salts in water softeners, which are literally contributing to the destruction of our fresh water supplies. Every time a water softener regenerates, each unit dumps twenty-five to one hundred pounds of salt into the local water supply. This can add up to a couple of tons per household annually in some locations! Salt doesn't "go away," so the salt levels keep going up in our water supplies.

HOW DO YOU MAKE WATER "WETTER"?

ACCORDING TO VAN Lue, the EPS unit that he developed charges the water with clouds of free electrons, which surround any dissolved solids in the water. This neutralizes these particles so they will have no chemical or electrostatic attraction to pipes, appliances or hot water heater elements. It also lowers the surface tension of the water by breaking the hydrogen bonding between the water molecules. This essentially makes the water "wetter."

The technology has been shown to produce a 30 percent to tenfold increase in plant growth and crop yield per acre when it is used for agricultural purposes. The ESP technology was taken to Saudi Arabia to help people there with their polluted water. The people were able to grow crops with water that is normally rated at between 5,000 to 6,000 parts sodium per million. In other words, the untreated water there contains so much salt and concentrated minerals that it will kill any crop with which it comes into contact. With the ESP units, farmers there have been able to raise crops that produced higher yields than they have ever seen using standard "sweet water" (classified as any water containing less than 500 parts per million of salt and minerals).

WE'RE EMULATING GOD'S METHODS

ONE OF THE advantages to the reverse-osmosis or distillation method of water purification is that it does more than merely filter water through carbon blocks or any other filtration system. Reverse osmosis, and to a lesser degree distillation, vitalizes the water. The process is similar to that which happens in the atmosphere through the interaction of electrostatic charges and high oxygen content. In the wild, animals would rather drink oxygenated water—even if it is muddy water in a ditch. Essentially, we are trying to emulate God's methods of sending rain through the atmosphere with our systems of reverse osmosis and distillation. Why? Oxygen is what gives water its taste, while minerals provide the aftertaste.

Fred's company also makes a unique shower filter that screws right onto the end of any standard shower pipe. It is totally portable for people who have to travel and stay in hotels a lot, so they can keep heavily chlorinated water from contaminating their skin. This is one of the most popular and affordable devices available, so I asked Fred to describe it:

> I found that most of the shower filters on the market use a substance called KDF, a zinc-copper composite, that knocks chlorine down very well. It also helps to reduce lead, but it doesn't remove the dangerous chlorine by-products, trichloromethanes, nor will it remove pesticides, herbicides or insecticides.
>
> We worked with some wonderful engineers to develop a filter that uses a modified KDF and more. Instead of using granular KDF (which bonds to itself and forms a lump that must be replaced very quickly), we had it spun into something similar to steel wool, only it *looks* like gold.
>
> The water runs through a channel of KDF wool first, then we send it through an exclusive filter containing more than 80 cubic inches of activated coconut shell carbon, which effectively removes all the chlorine by-products and chemicals. The filter lasts up to three years in many communities [other types claim to last a year, but have to be replaced after three months in some commu-

nities]. It is fully compatible with the standard half-inch shower pipe. There is a multimillion-dollar company that requires our filters be retrofitted to every hotel guest room whenever they bring their top executives into town for a meeting. They feel it's that important for their health.[5]

Most people who install a good quality shower filter will immediately notice a difference in the way their hair and skin feel and look. Many have written or called to say that within a week, other people were beginning to notice the change in their appearance.

One of the most important but predictable by-products of a good quality water filter (vs. one of the poorer quality varieties) in the kitchen area is a noticeable increase in the amount of water everyone is drinking. Families who begin to purify their water for the first time often give us dramatic testimonials. The reason is that most people without true water purification systems rarely drink tap water—and for good reason. It tastes so bad that they were drinking sodas and other acid-producing drinks just to escape the stuff coming out of the tap.

"THIS STUFF IS TOXIC!"

WHEN PARENTS TELL me, "Well, my kids don't want to drink the water because it tastes so bad," I tell them their kids are smarter than they realize. In reality, their bodies are telling them that the stuff is toxic, and they don't want to put it in their body! That water is often loaded with fluoride, chlorine, trichloromethanes, lead, arsenic, mercury and everything else that can seep into supplies from nearby landfills, dumps, factories and farmlands. Their body chemistry instinctively senses that. Unfortunately, those same senses can be fooled by heavy doses of sugar, flavoring and other stuff that mask many of the same chemicals and compounds in sodas and junk food. Adding ice to your drinking water can also numb your body's natural defense systems.

Take the poison test for me: Get yourself a nice glassful of chlorine-filled tap water *at room temperature.* Hold it up to your nose so you can get the full aroma of fresh processing chemicals and chlorine. Right about that time I guarantee that your body will be telling you, "Uh-oh, don't drink that—it's poison." Ignore the warning just this once. Hold your nose, bring it up to your lips and take a sip— just enough to roll around in your mouth. This time your taste buds will get into the act and tell you, "Stop! Don't drink this! It will poison you."

Then you can spit it out and order yourself a good quality water purifier!

Do yourself and your body a favor: Drink plenty of pure water every single day. Don't settle for anything less than the best, because you deserve it. It is one of the best "prescriptions" you can give yourself, and it will help every single cell in your body. Water is God's elixir of life; it is the most basic need of every living person on this planet. Water is a priority for life. Drink it pure, drink it often and drink at least half of your body weight in ounces daily. For more information on the products I have mentioned, please call my office at (800) 726-1834.

I BELIEVE THAT NO
SINGLE FACTOR PLAYS
A MORE SIGNIFICANT
ROLE IN THE ORIGIN
OF DISEASE——OR
IN ITS CURE OR
PREVENTION——THAN
OBTAINING SUFFICIENT
DIETARY FIBER.

Four

NATURAL FIBER—
CRUCIAL TO HEALTH
AND ENERGY

ADMIT IT: YOU aren't really excited about this chapter, are you? When was the last time you were drawn to the television set to watch a gripping special on dietary fiber and its effect on the colon? You can probably count on one hand the times "natural fiber" has entered your conversations in social settings (and you probably did your best to make a hasty retreat from that discussion, too). When doing my live seminars, I'll often ask the crowd for a show of hands concerning my topic of discussion. I *never ask* for a show of hands when it comes to the topic of constipation.

If it is true, and you are constipated, *I can absolutely guarantee you that your overall health and energy levels will improve* if you read this chapter all the way through and put my recommendations to the test! How can I make such a claim? Twenty years of research during which I have examined the nutritional aspects of hundreds of key illnesses, diseases and chronic health problems affecting Americans brought me to this startling conclusion. I am also convinced that no other single health condition plays so great a role in the development of disease as does *constipation.*

Constipation has been shown to have a role in the development of hemorrhoids, heart disease, atherosclerosis, cancer (too many types to mention), diabetes, gall bladder disease, kidney stones and ulcers—just to name a few. We know that dietary fiber helps to eliminate constipation without side effects, so why are so many Americans plagued by constipation to some degree or another? Usually it is because we simply do not get enough dietary fiber in the foods we eat day after day. The human digestive system, particularly the large intestine and colon, become constipated when too little dietary fiber and water are consumed.

There is no question that we do not consume nearly enough dietary fiber in America, and our digestive systems are severely "backed up" because of it. V. E. Irons, arguably the world's authority on colon hygiene, has stated that the U.S. Public Health Service has estimated that 90 percent of all Americans have a clogged colon to some degree![1]

The American Dietetic Association and the American Cancer Society have recommended that

we consume from 25 to 30 grams of fiber *daily.*
Many of the people I have counseled admitted to
me that they had trouble consuming 30 grams of
fiber a *week!*

What Is Fiber?

FIBER IS SIMPLY the part of your food that your
digestive system cannot break down and digest.
Your parents or grandparents probably called it
"roughage" or "bulk." Many people today associate
fiber only with bran (the outer husk of most types
of grain). Dietary fiber is most abundant in plant
products such as fruits, grains and vegetables. The
majority of the typical bowel movement consists of
fiber. (If it doesn't, stand by for difficulty and possibly even pain.)

There are two forms of fiber, soluble and insoluble fiber. Soluble fiber such as pectin (found in
most fruits) dissolves easily in water so it can be
absorbed in the intestine and circulated in the
blood stream. Soluble fiber in the blood has the
ability to attach itself to blood fats and create a
complex that will remove these fats from the blood
system, thus lowering cholesterol.

Insoluble fiber absorbs water also, but it is not
absorbed in the intestine. It remains there and
forms the majority of the bulk necessary to "sweep"
bodily wastes through the intestine and out of the

body. Without this fiber, food waste and bodily processes move very slowly through the colon (if at all). This abnormally slow-moving mass can putrefy or rot right in the body!

SHOW ME THE BRAN

I AM OFTEN asked, "How much is 25 grams of fiber, and where can I get it?" One serving of bran flakes contains about 4 grams of fiber, and a large unpeeled apple contains approximately 3 to 4 grams of fiber. (The things Americans eat the most—processed foods like pasta, most breads, meats, dairy products and most junk food—contain no fiber at all!)

To make sure you consume enough fiber, I recommend that you eat a breakfast centered around high fiber every day. Then eat at least five servings of fresh fruit and vegetables daily in accordance with the recommendations of the American Cancer Society. You may also take a fiber supplement several times a week. I use oat bran and psyllium on a regular basis.

You will probably avoid constipation altogether if you include this amount of fiber in your daily diet. Constipation is largely a phenomenon unique to Western civilization. In our "wisdom," we process out most of the nutrients and bran that occur naturally in our wheat, rice, corn and other grains. Then we eat what is left.

It is ironic that by carefully "refining" our wheat, we remove over fifty nutrients in the process. Then we add twelve synthetic vitamins (many of them petroleum-based formulations that are totally indigestible), proudly label the stuff as "enriched" and boldly claim in national advertising that it is healthy to eat. What a culture we have in America! Who else would throw away what is nutritious and eat what is not? The part that is left over after processing is basically a "glue ball" waiting to happen. Nearly everyone in America is constipated—whether they know it or not.

ANYTHING BUT "REGULAR"

I ASKED ONE woman who came into my office if she had any problems with irregularity or constipation. She said, "No, I am very regular. *I have a bowel movement every Thursday.*" I realize that bowel movements vary from person to person, but this dear woman was anything but "regular." (I once knew a woman in Tallahassee, Florida, who had a bowel movement only once a month when she started her period. Her health was a wreck, and she was always sick.)

The truth is that fecal matter is bodily waste. That woman ate three full meals, or one to five pounds of food per day, but she only disposed of her bodily "garbage" once a week. What do you think that waste did inside her body? Everyone should have two or three bowel movements daily. This helps any waste matter to move quickly through the large intestine and colon. "Transit time" is the time period measured from the time we eat our food to the time all the waste products from the same meal are finally eliminated. This transit time should be no more than twenty-four hours (ideally, less than eighteen hours).

Medical treatment of uncomplicated constipation generally consists of increasing dietary fiber, drinking more water and moderate exercise. A report in the *Journal of the American Medical Society* recommended that patients who are chronically constipated (the "regular" lady who moved her bowels every Thursday would definitely qualify as "chronically constipated") gradually increase their daily bran consumption from ½ cup to 1½ cups of bran daily (27 grams).[2] A second study noted specifically that oat bran is superior to wheat and corn bran in its ability to lower blood fats, making it obviously desirable.[3]

Although medical doctors agree on the need for regular elimination of bodily wastes, many of them still advise their patients suffering from constipation to take over-the-counter chemical laxatives. These laxatives purge whatever is in the colon and force it out, but they are very harsh on the system.

Many are habit forming. Sometimes doctors will prescribe a "bulk laxative" to relieve constipation. Bulk laxatives are not chemical products; they simply provide the missing fiber needed to form a bowel movement.

DAILY BRAN KEEPS THINGS MOVING

ONE STUDY COMPARED the effectiveness of these bulk laxatives with that of simple bran in treating geriatric patients suffering from chronic constipation. The report found that bran supplementation provided relief, or bowel movement, 30 percent faster than did the bulk laxative. The report also suggested that daily bran supplementation beginning at an early age could prevent constipation altogether.[4]

You might appreciate something else that dietary fiber can do for you. There is a one-in-three chance that you are suffering from hemorrhoids right now, even as you are reading these words. If you are over the age of fifty, then there is a 50 percent chance you are in this group of silent sufferers.[5] The way you could "spell relief" is most likely *d-i-e-t-a-r-y f-i-b-e-r.*

Hemorrhoids aren't very pleasant to talk about, but they are even more unpleasant to live with! They are perhaps one of the most common plagues of our Western culture, and *they are often caused by constipation and a low-fiber diet.* You are probably beginning to see a pattern here, which is exactly what I have been hoping for.

Just inside the rectum and anus (the opening where fecal material leaves the body) are the anal cushions, or folds in the tissues of the digestive tract. These folds are filled with numerous blood veins and other tissue. (Veins, which bring blood back to the heart after it has been used by the cells of the body, have thinner walls than arteries, which take freshly oxygenated blood from the heart and distribute it to the body.) When these veins become swollen or enlarged, they can actually bulge into finger-like projections of tissue that literally protrude into the buttocks or rectum. These swollen and enlarged veins are called *hemorrhoids,* and they can cause pain, discomfort, burning and itching that is severe enough to make everyday living all but unbearable.

BIG-LEAGUE HEMORRHOIDS

HEMORRHOIDS MADE THE prime-time news several years ago when George Brett, then the star shortstop for the Kansas City Royals professional baseball team, underwent surgery to relieve his discomfort with hemorrhoids and had to sit out some games. The very nature of this problem makes it a natural source of humor and snickering, but those who are suffering from the pain and itching of hemorrhoids are anything but amused. Hemorrhoids can lead to the more serious problem of rectal bleeding, which in turn can lead to other more serious problems associated with chronic and acute blood loss.

Hemorrhoids are sometimes caused by genetic factors or by increased venous pressure in the anus and rectum. Several factors can contribute to this increased pressure, including constipation, straining to force a bowel movement, obesity, pregnancy, sitting or standing for long periods of time or heavy lifting. Of all these factors, constipation and the low intake of dietary fiber appear to be the most consistent hemorrhoid-causing factors among Americans. This becomes even more evident when you consider the fact that hemorrhoids are almost unheard of in countries where high-fiber, unrefined foods are dietary staples.[6]

When a patient seeks medical help for uncomplicated hemorrhoids, he or she will probably leave the appointment with a list of prescribed treatments identical to the home remedies available to any consumer at the local drug store. (Please note that this book in no way seeks to diagnose or prescribe any specific therapeutic regimen for any condition. While anyone can purchase the products listed in this book, we maintain that all medical conditions and treatments should be discussed with a qualified physician.)

As noted earlier, the initial treatment for hemorrhoids and the constipation that often causes them generally begins with a gradual increase of dietary fiber. In fact, according to an article reported in *American Family Physician,* a journal designed for family physicians, dietary fiber is considered the *mainstay* of treatment for hemorrhoids.[7] Studies have shown that when fiber supplements were added to the diet of hemorrhoid sufferers, they experienced a significant improvement in their symptoms—including the reduction of pain, itching and rectal bleeding during bowel movements.[8]

DIETARY FIBER REDUCES HARDENING OF THE ARTERIES

THE INCREASED INTAKE of dietary fiber, along with cleaning out the colon, has been clinically shown to reduce atherosclerosis, also known as hardening of the arteries. This is the process whereby cholesterol and fats in the blood build up on artery walls and eventually clog them. In the latter stages of this disease, blood flow to an area of the body can become totally blocked. If this happens around the heart, the result is a myocardial infarction—a type of heart attack. In the vasculature of the brain, atherosclerosis may lead to stroke.

There is no doubt or question that this process of atherosclerosis is related to the high-saturated-fat, low-fiber diet of our Western culture. The goal in the treatment or prevention of atherosclerosis is to lower the level of fats in the blood—a process in which fiber can play an important role. Fiber has the unique ability to bond with dietary fats and cholesterol in the digestive system and to transform them into a complex that cannot be absorbed in the digestive tract (that means they cannot be transferred to the blood either). The fat and cholesterol then become fecal material and are eliminated relatively quickly with defecation, thus *lowering total levels of dietary fat and cholesterol in the blood.*

Experimental studies have shown that soluble fiber supplementation with products such as oats, barley, pectin (found in fruits and vegetables) and alfalfa significantly reduce serum (blood) cholesterol levels. Another study conducted with nondiabetic patients with elevated serum cholesterol demonstrated the same thing. Pectin, a soluble fiber found in most fruits, was proven to decrease total levels of cholesterol in just a short period of time!

In one experiment, patients were able to significantly lower their cholesterol *in just one month* by eating two to three apples a day. Grapefruit pectin, considered by some to be the best source of cholesterol-lowering pectin, has been shown to have a specificity for binding to harmful blood fats.[9] It gets even better. Another experimental study gave patients 15 grams of citrus pectin daily for three weeks. These patients lowered their cholesterol by 13 percent while increasing the amount of fats eliminated in their bowel movements by 44 percent![10]

DIETARY FIBER HELPS PREVENT CANCER

THE AMERICAN CANCER Society has stated publicly that a high-fiber diet can help prevent some forms of cancer. Research has clearly shown that a high-fiber diet offers protection from cancer of the colon, prostate and breast. In women, risk factors for breast cancer include early onset menarche and a *high-fat diet,* both of which can increase levels of the female hormone estrogen, which is known to act like "fertilizer" to some forms of breast cancer. Fiber can even assist in the excretion of excess levels of estrogen![11]

Other studies examining the incidence of colon cancer and diet have clearly shown a correlation between a high-fat, low-fiber diet (which is typical of Western nations) and colon cancer.[12] On the positive side, international comparison studies in nations where a *high-fiber diet* is a way of life have shown that colon and rectal cancers in these countries are very rare. These studies clearly suggest that eating a variety of high-fiber foods will offer protection from colon cancer.[13] Other studies have also shown that increasing fiber intake can decrease the risk of prostate cancer in men.[14]

HIGH-FIBER DIETS HELP CONTROL BLOOD SUGAR LEVELS

WITH GROWING NUMBERS of Americans being diagnosed with diabetes milletus or some other blood sugar disorder every year, wouldn't you like to hear some good news about preventive measures in this area? Believe it or not, high-fiber diets have also been proven to be helpful in the control of blood sugar levels in patients with diabetes, especially the adult-onset form of the disease (the most common form). In one study where patients were placed on a high-fiber diet for three months, *all* the participants experienced significant improvement in glucose maintenance and decreases in body fats.[15] Other researchers have suggested that a high-fiber diet can actually lead to improvement in the diabetic's condition to the point that many will be able to decrease or even eliminate their need for diabetic medications![16]

Hypertension, or high blood pressure, is another disease process directly associated with the Western high-fat, low-fiber diet and sedentary lifestyle.

Although the role of fiber in the pathogenesis and treatment of hypertension is not completely clear, researchers have repeatedly shown the benefits of increasing fiber in the diets of patients with high blood pressure. In one study, researchers were so confident that they went to a health food store and found three hundred volunteers. These shoppers, who were not necessarily high blood pressure patients, each had their blood pressure measured. Following this they were placed on a diet that increased their dietary fiber by 100 grams a week. Researchers soon found what they had suspected: Even healthy volunteers experienced a reduction in their blood pressure with increased dietary fiber.[17]

Another study involved volunteers at the other end of the health spectrum. This experiment took diabetic men who also had elevated blood pressure (a very common complication of diabetes) and placed them on a high-fiber diet. Amazingly, in just *two weeks,* these men had an average 10 percent drop in their blood pressure![18] Numerous other studies confirm the results of these two studies.[19]

Dietary fiber is especially important if you are trying to lose weight wisely (while avoiding the countless numbers of "diet fads" plaguing the American public). It is absolutely critical that you make sure that you have two or three bowel movements every single day. Many people who have problems with constipation also have problems with excess body weight. It is often because their digestive systems are so sluggish.

You can easily become depressed if you have a big meal and the food just stays in your system for two or three days. Every time you step on the weight scales, it will say you have gained four extra pounds—even though you really haven't gained that weight. You have basically pressed that food weight into your intestinal tract, and it hasn't cleared your system yet. Many people battle depression and frustration over this unending cycle of discouragement—and it isn't made any easier by the terrible way they feel.

Several years ago, I read a report that stated when medical examiners autopsied the body of a well-known singer after his untimely death, they discovered that his colon weighed sixty pounds! It was speculated that it weighed that much because he had become so obese and was having problems with constipation. The colon is an elastic organ that will actually expand and open up to incredible proportions when necessary. In fact, some people who have been autopsied had colons that measured nine inches in diameter (while normally it is only two inches in diameter)! These oversized organs contribute to obesity along with a host of other conditions. It is really unhealthy to live under the strain of chronic constipation, and it is needless.

The solution to this serious health problem is only one healthy food choice away.

THE VALUE OF "COLONIC CLEANSING"

MANY PEOPLE HAVE found tremendous relief by combining a high-fiber supplementation program with a colonic cleansing program. Many physicians turned their nose up at the colonic irrigation procedure with the advent of the synthetic laxative, preferring to write a prescription rather than deal with the difficulty and "mess" of this therapeutic procedure. Unlike an enema, which only flushes out the first twelve inches of the colon, a true colonic irrigation will gently cleanse the entire length of the colon. I have worked with many people who have gone through colonic cleansing programs and have seen some miraculous results. Please call my office at (800) 726-1834 for more details.

The importance of a high-fiber, low-fat diet becomes even more significant when you realize that cardiovascular disease was virtually unheard of a hundred years ago in this country! Rampant heart and circulatory disease is a phenomenon of this century and began when we started milling our grains and removing vitamin E and natural fiber out of our food. It is interesting to note that of the top ten risk factors that lead to cardiovascular death, seven are *directly related to diet.*

A diet rich in dietary fiber goes a long, long way toward restoring and maintaining premium function of your cardiovascular system, your blood glucose levels and your blood pressure levels. Doesn't it make a lot of sense to prevent disease by making wise choices at the dinner table today, instead of treating some debilitating disease tomorrow with expensive, dangerous and intrusive medical procedures on the operating table or hospital bed? Next time you come to the table, say, "Pass the fruit and vegetables and fiber supplement, please." It's a decision you can live with!

NUTRITIONAL DEFICIENCY DISEASES IN HUMANS HELPED US TO DISCOVER MANY OF OUR VITAMIN AND MINERAL REQUIREMENTS—EVEN BEFORE WE KNEW THERE WERE VITAMINS.

Five

SUPPLEMENT YOUR DIET WITH VITAMINS (ESPECIALLY THOSE VITAL ANTIOXIDANTS)

URING THE LATE seventeenth and early eighteenth centuries, virtually every crew member aboard sea-going sailing vessels on long voyages away from land was affected by scurvy—but only after crew members' stores of fresh fruits and vegetables were depleted. Scurvy caused spongy gums, loosening of the teeth and bleeding into the skin and mucous membranes. The need for ascorbic acid (vitamin C) was discovered when sailors noticed that fresh citrus fruits such as lemons and limes and certain leafy vegetables cured or totally prevented these symptoms. Their problems cleared up very quickly once the crew members had access to fresh fruits, vegetables or other foods containing ascorbic acid (vitamin C).

During my pursuit of one of my degrees from Florida State University, I was required to conduct animal research as part of my study. I remain convinced that the vast majority of animal experimentation are unnecessary, but I noticed that test animals in the university labs were routinely fed very nutritious food. The reason was very simple: If they didn't have a nutritious menu, many of the animals would die of "deficiency diseases" before any experiments could be conducted or completed.

Nutritional deficiency diseases in humans helped us to discover many of our vitamin and mineral requirements—even before we knew there were vitamins. Research labs revealed that human beings require about ninety essential vitamins, minerals and trace minerals every single day for optimum health. If we don't get these nutrients in sufficient concentrations, we can develop serious deficiency diseases and die prematurely.

Your body requires certain nutrients for proper health and function. You need approximately sixty different minerals, sixteen vitamins, twelve amino acids and three essential fatty acids every day. (The reason I say approximate is because many of the so-called "experts" can't even agree on this number.) If those nutrients *are not supplied by the food you eat* or through some other means such as vitamin supplementation, then you *will* have health problems. The nutritional needs of animals are very similar, especially among mammals. A good dog food will contain around forty essential minerals, while a good rat food will contain around twenty-eight minerals. Sadly, I have never found a *human infant baby formula that contains even close to this many minerals!* If newborns have to have these minerals and they are fed by formula, where are they supposed to get these nutrients? Is it a coincidence that some researchers are now linking human infant formula to childhood diabetes and other types of disorders? Also, did you know that in the United States, the leading cause of death in children other than accidents is cancer? The United States has the highest infant death rate of any industrialized society. Do you think that just maybe infant formula may be involved?

Isn't Good Food Good Enough?

MANY PEOPLE SAY to me, "I get everything I need from the food that I eat; there is no way I need to take vitamins or supplements." I am convinced there is absolutely no way you can receive all the nutrients you need from the food you eat given the mineral-deficient state of America's farm lands today. It is literally *impossible.* The soil doesn't have the nutrients, so the plants can't either.

The agricultural industry does a lot of things to increase yield-per-acre figures, but those things don't necessarily increase the quality of the food produced (and eaten by American consumers).

Our bodies need nearly ninety nutrients, but the average farm field generally receives only nitrogen, phosphorous and potassium to increase its crop yield. Unfortunately, these soil additives do nothing to replace the minerals lost through modern farming techniques. Five or ten years of continuous growing seasons will pretty much deplete all the trace minerals normally present in good farmland such as zinc, boron, tin, copper, selenium and calcium. (Again, the Bible tells us to allow the fields to rest. You'll be amazed when you start digging at how much practical information the "Good Book" contains.)

My paternal grandfather lived to be ninety-one years old. My maternal grandfather lived to be eighty-six years old. Neither man took vitamins or supplements, so if what I am saying is true, then how did they live so long? Both of my grandfathers were born in the 1800s, and they ate fresh, farm-grown food from fields that were routinely rotated and fertilized with natural manure fertilizer.

The trace minerals in those fields were replaced every year, so there were a lot of minerals and nutrients in their food. They picked their home-grown vegetables and fruits when they were ripe and ate them within the hour in most cases. Today, most of the vegetables and fruits in our grocery stores are picked while still green (and low in nutrients), then shipped hundreds or thousands of miles to an agricultural holding house where they are immersed in different types of gases to make them ripen prematurely. This explains why you have to sort through a display of oranges to find an *orange* orange for your children. (If you look closely at the label, you may see a notice stating that the fruit has been treated with gas.) Also remember there weren't thousands of synthetic chemicals and pesticides used on the food in the 1800s.

THE CASE FOR VITAMINS

ANYONE WHO IS serious about preventing disease by making wise food choices and consistently supplementing their diet with vitamin supplements should be prepared for an uphill battle. Although research continues to substantiate the value of vitamin supplements for the human body, many medical doctors still believe they are unnecessary. Yet, although the United States is blessed with some of the most highly trained, dedicated and conscientious medical professionals in the world, the life expectancy for medical doctors in the U.S. is around fifty-eight years—while the life expectancy of other Americans averages between seventy-two to seventy-four years of age.

Most of the doctors in this nation have never been trained in the area of nutrition or nutritional supplementation. Dr. John McDougall noted in

The McDougall Plan that medical schools tend to overlook nutrition in their curriculum:

> A recent investigation of a Senate subcommittee revealed that the average physician in the United States receives less than three hours of training in nutrition during four years of medical school and that less than 3 percent of the licensing exam questions are concerned with nutrition. Because of this deficiency in training, few doctors will understand or encourage any interest you may express in nutrition.[1]

I am happy, however, to report that every doctor I've met who had received nutritional training or who took the trouble to research the facts about nutrient supplementation has become positive about it. These informed physicians all suggest to their patients that they use vitamins and minerals on a regular basis.

VERY CHEAP INSURANCE

PROFESSIONAL HEALTH ASSOCIATIONS tend to follow the leader, whether right or wrong. The American Dietetic Association has stated publicly that "the best nutritional strategy for promoting optimal health and reducing the risk of chronic disease is to obtain adequate nutrients from a wide variety of foods." They recommend vitamin supplements only as a second alternative.[2] However, I found that when I personally interviewed individual members of this association, nearly all of them admitted that they take daily vitamin supplements! Frankly, I would rather spend a dollar a day for vitamin supplements than believe the naysayers. Basically, the use of vitamins is very, very cheap health insurance. I'll take the "expensive urine" on the chance that good nutrition will extend my length and quality of life rather than end up with diseases spawned by nutritional deficiencies and die at the age of fifty-eight.

In September 1993, the National Cancer Institute and Harvard University issued an "anti-cancer diet" based on a five-year study conducted in China. Researchers tracked a group of twenty-nine thousand people over the five-year period and discovered that when they supplemented the diets of the test subjects, the vitamin supplementation appeared to be responsible for a 9 percent reduction of death overall (from all causes). Even more significant was the 13 percent reduction of cancer in the group, with an amazing 21 percent reduction of stomach and esophageal cancers (the primary problems being studied). The target group was given consistent supplements of vitamin E, beta carotene and selenium.[3]

You have probably never heard about that land-mark study, and I am not surprised. We are no closer to finding a cure for cancer today than we were forty years ago, despite the billions of dollars that have been spent in traditional medical research. The only hope we have is in learning how to *prevent* the disease. I wish we would pay attention to the very studies that have been conducted. Unfortunately, there appears to be a blind spot where nutritional solutions to physical problems are concerned.

VITAMINS AND ANTIOXIDANTS: HOW MUCH AND WHY

VITAMINS ARE ORGANIC substances that are essential to the nutrition of most animals and some plants. Our bodies need only minute quantities of these substances to help regulate key metabolic processes necessary for life. The human body can manufacture certain vitamins, but it extracts most of its vitamin needs from the foods we eat and, in the modern era, from dietary vitamin and mineral supplements.

We have known about antioxidants since the early 1900s, but today they are coming into their own. More than twenty thousand articles per year have been published on the interaction between free radicals and antioxidants. Twenty years ago we talked to people about nutrition and health and made special emphasis about the need for antioxidants in our diets, but no one was interested. There has been a traditional mindblock that resists acknowledging any correlation between what we eat and how healthy we are (usually because *knowledge* demands *change*).

It is time to acknowledge the truth, especially in this day. Previous generations didn't have to feed their children products produced by a food industry that uses five thousand to seven thousand chemical food additives to "enhance" the Jonathan apple on the teacher's desk, the birthday cake you ordered for your oldest child and the Thanksgiving turkey in Grandma's oven.

WELCOME TO THE MODERN ERA

MANY OF OUR modern diseases were virtually unknown to previous generations, leading researchers to believe they are caused by elements unique to our modern culture. Alum, the source of aluminum, is abundant in nature, but it takes on different characteristics once it is processed into the light metal that is so prevalent in modern societies. Alzheimer's disease appears to be one of the "modern plagues" primarily seen only in our generation. Since aluminum may be a culprit in the global epidemic of Alzheimer's disease, I along with many other natural health practitioners believe that the sale of aluminum pots and pans needs to be eliminated globally. Have you ever noticed that the aluminum pans you use on a regular basis pit? Well, where do you think this aluminum goes? Obviously into your food. Avoid as much as possible any exposure to this mineral.

When studies based on autopsies of Alzheimer's patients showed that some of the victims had abnormally high levels of aluminum in their brain tissues, for the first time people began to see just how much this metal has infiltrated their lives. We cook in aluminum pots and pans and store our leftovers in aluminum foil. We drink sodas out of aluminum cans, and we've abandoned simple deodorants in favor of more convenient antiperspirants, which use aluminum chlorhydrate. Nearly every kitchen in American contains boxes and canisters holding powdered components such as baking powder and table salt—along with a little-known anticoagulation agent called aluminum triscillate. We consume incredible amounts of tasty antacid tablets daily, not realizing that many of them contain unhealthy levels of aluminum salts.

People are beginning to accept the idea that in most cases their level of health rises and falls over time with the patterns of what they eat and drink every day. Given the poor nutritional quality of much of the food eaten by this generation, we start the race for health with a serious handicap. Even the most cynical among us are now admitting that we can no longer get away with drinking a fifth of whiskey—or eating a pound of bacon—every day for the next twenty-five years and still live to be seventy-five years old.

UNENDING MOLECULAR WARS

OUR BODIES WAGE a life-and-death battle every moment of our lives, whether we are asleep or awake. It is the battle between excessive free radicals and the antioxidants in our bodies, and it takes place at the molecular level.

In his book *The Antioxidant Revolution,* Dr. Kenneth H. Cooper says that we can decrease our risk of heart disease, atherosclerosis and cancer by using the key antioxidants—vitamin E, vitamin C and beta carotene—in association with consistent exercise and healthy eating habits. Dr. Cooper helped America's first astronauts prepare for the rigors of space travel, then he sounded the exercise alarm in 1968 and alerted the nation to the dangers of the sedentary lifestyle. He introduced the American public to aerobic exercise and launched a revolution in fitness with his first book, *Aerobics,* which many credit with increasing the nation's level of cardiovascular health.

Every breathing thing on this planet needs

oxygen to survive. But human beings can get "too much of a good thing" where oxygen is concerned. Dr. Cooper described the dilemma this way in *The Antioxidant Revolution:*

> Most of the oxygen we breathe is stable and essential to our health and well-being. Other unstable oxygen molecules—which include the free radicals and their kin—may also behave in ways that are good for us. But on occasion, the radicals may turn into the classic case of good guys gone bad.[4]

OUR BODIES MANUFACTURE CERTAIN ANTIOXIDANTS

UNDER IDEAL CONDITIONS without the environmental hazards and health-poor lifestyles common to our generation, our bodies would probably manufacture enough antioxidants internally to keep excess free radicals under control. The truth is that we do not live under ideal conditions, and we do not get enough vitamins, minerals or antioxidants from our diets. That means we need diet supplementation.

After noting that free radicals have been solidly linked to heart and blood vessel disease, cancer, cataracts and the breakdown of body tissues common to aging, Dr. Cooper said the list of additional diseases linked to free radicals reads "like the index of a medical encyclopedia," including more than fifty medical conditions such as stroke, asthma, pancreatitis, inflammatory bowel disease, Parkinson's disease, leukemia and high blood pressure.[5]

To properly understand a *free radical,* we will have to touch briefly on some biochemistry concepts. The common water molecule, H_2O, is two hydrogen atoms bonded to one oxygen atom. These atoms are bonded together very tightly through differences in their electrical charge. Normal chemical reactions in the body can force this molecule to split into two unequal parts—one oxygen and hydrogen combination (OH) and a solitary hydrogen atom (H).

These parts of the original water molecule are now unstable because their electrical properties are unstable or unbalanced. They are now "free radicals" with a driving need to regain a neutral electrical balance. They do this by "stealing" electrons or atoms, or by bonding themselves where they do not belong. At the cellular level in the human body, free radicals will steal atoms or protons from the various cells of the body, causing cell injury and possibly altering the cell's DNA with deadly consequences.

Beware the Cellular Wrecking Crews

To complicate matters, the antioxidants we manufacture in our bodies are easily overcome when excess amounts of free radicals are released through the effects of environmental and lifestyle factors such as cigarette smoking, pollution, drugs, ultraviolet light, pesticides, radiation, emotional stress, asbestos, joint tissue injuries and sore or strained muscles.

Dr. Cooper described the dangerous side of free radicals when their aggressive characteristics operate outside of proper boundaries:

> As a result of their instability, free radicals are constantly on the lookout for other molecules they can lock on to, like little magnets. (At times, radicals are referred to as "cellular wrecking crews" because of the damage they inflict after they combine with another molecule.) They exist alone for only a fleeting microsecond before they smash into another molecule.[6]

Call in the Good Guys

Your body manufactures three "endogenous" or "homemade" antioxidants: super oxide dismuitase (SOD), catalase and glutathione peroxidase

(GSH). These antioxidants would do a pretty good job of controlling wayward free radicals in a safer, saner world. But there are too many environmental and lifestyle variables releasing clouds of free radicals in our bodies for the "homeboys" to handle alone. Exercise and proper food choices can help strengthen our internal antioxidant resources, but we still need to supplement our diets with "exogenus" or outside antioxidants to help scavenge and neutralize free radicals. Dr. Cooper calls the three primary antioxidants—vitamin E, vitamin C and beta carotene—"the Antioxidant Marines."[7]

Dr. Dean Ornish also says that this antioxidant trio works together, "acting as scavengers of free-radical molecules that can harm your DNA, your genetic blueprint, helping to prevent cancer. Also, they can help prevent cholesterol from being changed into a form that is more likely to deposit in your arteries."[8]

VITAMIN E: NATURE'S BLOOD THINNER

VITAMIN E IS absolutely critical to human health because it acts as an antiplaquing agent in the blood and helps to prevent atherosclerotic plaquing. If your doctor is thinking of placing you on a blood-thinning medication, talk with him about placing you on a good natural vitamin E source first for a reasonable trial period. The World

Health Organization claims that *a lack of vitamin E in the diet* is the number one reason so many people in this country (and internationally) die of heart disease![9]

Vitamin E also helps to preserve and strengthen the immune system function and has been shown to be beneficial in the fight against cancer.[10] It helps reduce the levels of nitrosamines and other cancer-causing substances found in the stool.[11] Vitamin E also appears to inhibit the growth of some forms of cancer cells.[12]

I recommend that you take about 800 International Units of vitamin E every day.

If you increase your oxygen intake by 20 percent (which is pretty easy to do if you start an aerobics class, begin a vigorous exercise routine or participate in strenuous athletic competition) then your body will also be forming extra free radicals. I recommend that you take at least 1200 International Units of natural vitamin E every day that you exercise strenuously.

By the way, Dr. Kenneth Cooper's research on free radicals confirmed that synthetic vitamin E does not work. (Synthetic vitamin E is made out of petroleum or turpentine in most cases.)

As a student at Florida State, I was taught that chemical vitamins were the same as natural vitamins, but when I started my practice in Florida nearly twenty years ago, I also discovered that synthetic vitamin supplements do not work. There is no such thing as a good "cheap" vitamin. When you go to a discount store and pick up a bottle of generic multiple vitamins for $1.29, you have probably just purchased a bottle of encapsulated petroleum extracts.

Years ago my clinic used to sell a little "Vitapac" containing samples of different vitamin supplements from a variety of manufacturers. We ran a test on these supplements by placing them in an oven and heating them to 200 degrees Fahrenheit. The supplements made from petroleum-based coal tar melted back down into petroleum distillates and coal tar, while the natural vitamins did not. I refuse to feed a vitamin made out of plastic or gasoline to a human being. It is like feeding someone a Crisco pill—it doesn't work. One of my dogs, an Alaskan malamute, snatched one of those Vitapaks one time. We were amazed when we realized that she had eaten all of the natural supplements while leaving the coal tar supplements on the floor.

If your doctor or health practitioner has placed you on anticoagulant therapy, make sure you consult with him or her before you take vitamin E supplements to avoid any problems or health complications.

VITAMIN C: THE HEALING ANTIOXIDANT

VITAMIN C PROMOTES wound healing, tissue repair and proper tissue growth. It also helps your body utilize iron, and it increases your body's immunity to infectious diseases. It has been shown to lower total blood cholesterol levels and raise the HDL (good) cholesterol. Vitamin C also enhances the effect of vitamin E in the body, and together the vitamins function as highly effective nitrite scavengers (nitrites are some of the most potent cancer-causing substances known).

One study demonstrated that the addition of 2,000 milligrams (2 grams) of vitamin C to the diet blocks the formation of the cancer-forming chemicals called *nitrosamines*, which have been positively linked to the development of colon cancer. This demonstrates that vitamin C provides a protective benefit against colon cancer.[13]

Vitamin C helps your body recover more quickly from injuries, sicknesses and fatigue. When combined with bioflavanoids, it helps strengthen capillary walls in the body. Many people suffer through cold after cold because of what they eat and because they have a deficiency of vitamin C. This vitamin is absolutely critical to proper cellular integrity, and it is one of the primary components of collagen. That is why people develop gum problems when their levels of vitamin C get low.

I generally recommend a daily supplement of 1,000 to 3,000 milligrams of vitamin C. Take a *minimum* of 1,000 milligrams three times per day if you exercise regularly. If cancer prevention is your primary goal due to family history or the presence of cancer in your body, I recommend a daily dose of 5,000 to 10,000 milligrams (5 to 10 grams) of vitamin C in buffered ascorbate form. I prefer powdered vitamin C ascorbate, because it is a *pH-neutral* form of ascorbic acid. Remember that vitamin C is ascorbic acid. If you get too much into your system, it can contribute to forcing your body chemistry into an acidic range, which is very unhealthy in itself.

Some people experience side effects such as loose bowels or gas when taking 1,000 milligrams or more of vitamin C per day, and a few report these symptoms while taking half that dosage. Most people report no problems, however, even at much higher dosages. If you have a history of kidney stones, you should consult with your doctor about your daily vitamin C intake. If you give your children a chewable form of vitamin C, make sure it is a pH-neutral product. If it is not pH-balanced, it may dissolve the calcium in your child's tooth enamel, because most forms of vitamin C are extremely acidic.

BETA CAROTENE:
THE STRESS AND CANCER BUSTER

BETA CAROTENE HELPS to reduce the risk of lung cancer, oral cancer, bladder cancer and rectal and skin tumors. Hundreds of scientific studies and research articles have shown that beta carotene reduces the risk of cancer. Beta carotene is a precursor to vitamin A. The body manufactures vitamin A from the beta carotene found in "yellow" fruits like cantaloupe and in vegetables such as sweet potatoes, as well as in green leafy vegetables.

Beta carotene seems to offer protection against lung cancer and cervical cancer. In one survey where six thousand people were studied, a definite link was found between low levels of beta carotene consumption and lung cancer.[14] According to the prestigious English medical journal *Lancet,* one study of 1,954 people conducted over a nineteen-year period also found that the lower the levels of beta carotene intake, the higher the incidence of lung cancer.[15] Women with cervical cancer have been shown to have significantly lower levels of beta carotene in their systems than do women with similar backgrounds who do not have the disease.[16] You should take supplemental beta carotene every single day.

ADDITIONAL VITAMIN SUPPLEMENTS OF VALUE

SELENIUM DEFICIENCIES HAVE been positively associated with cancer. In a study where cancer-causing agents were used to induce cancer in lab animals, those having selenium supplementation had at least 35 percent less incidence of contracting cancer![17] In another study of 4,480 adults, it was found that their risk of developing cancer could be predicted by the level of selenium in their blood, with low levels being high risk.[18]

Study after study has confirmed the cancer-protective benefits of selenium in many forms of cancer, including breast, skin, lung, colon, prostate and even leukemia cancers.[19] A disease called cardiomyopathy, commonly called "White Muscle Disease," is caused by selenium deficiency. Several famous sports figures were struck by this disease in recent years, and many of its victims must undergo heart transplants or die. Oddly enough, for about ten cents worth of selenium a day, this kind of condition can nearly always be prevented. I recommend that you take 200 micrograms of selenium per day.

Vitamin B₆ helps to remove excess water and helps you to feel better about yourself and look better almost immediately. I recommend that you take 15 milligrams three times a day. This supplement also helps women having problems with menopause and PMS. I recommend that women dealing with the discomfort of PMS take 50 milligrams one to two times a day.

Calcium and boron should be taken together. They help to produce the estrogen and testosterone hormones that regulate our sex drives and secondary physical characteristics. (Men who have boron deficiencies often have a problem with their sex drive or libido.)

Mike was a bodybuilder who was experiencing problems with kidney stones and prostitis. I told him, "Mike, if you are passing kidney stones, that means you may have a calcium deficiency. Calcium deficiencies are linked to more than a hundred different types of diseases." He did exactly what I told him to do, and within a few days he started having relief from the pain. He also had a lot more energy and felt a whole lot better.

People are always telling me, "I have kidney stones, so I have to limit my calcium intake." The exact opposite is true. Studies in recent years have shown that individuals eating diets rich in calcium have remained literally free of kidney stones.

Calcium deficiencies have been linked to more than 147 different types of diseases, including Bell's Palsy, osteoporosis, receding gum lines, high blood pressure, kidney stones, bone spurs, heel spurs, calcium deposits, cramps, twitches and PMS symptoms.

Calcium should always be combined with magnesium and boron for maximum absorption. I recommend 500 milligrams of calcium citrate per day.

Copper deficiency can increase your risk of ruptured aortic aneurysms, a loss of elasticity in the skin and the blood vessel walls, premature gray hair, wrinkling and varicose veins. Copper, like most trace minerals and metals, must be taken in a colloidal or plant-based form for proper digestion. The body needs very little copper for proper function, and too much will actually be toxic to the body. Our need for this element can generally be met through our diet. Supplementation should be limited to 2 milligrams daily.

Zinc deficiencies have been linked to the loss of the sense of smell and to a decrease in sperm count.

Other "rare-earth" trace minerals have actually doubled the life span of lab animals. Most of these trace minerals are readily available from "colloidal" or plant-based food sources that are easy to digest.

Iron is an essential nutrient that is readily available from unsulphured black strap molasses, which also contains many other important nutrients. Available at most health food stores, it raises the iron levels of pregnant women better than anything we've ever used in our office. We recommend taking at least a teaspoon of unsulphured black strap molasses every single day, especially if you are a woman and are still in your child-bearing years. (Do not use iron in tablet form; it has been linked to increased risks of heart disease.)

COLLOIDAL MINERAL SUPPLEMENTS ARE THE BEST

AVOID MINERAL SUPPLEMENTS such as oyster shell and dolomite, because these forms of calcium have only an 8 to 12 percent absorption rate if you are younger than forty, and only a 3 to 5 percent absorption after the age of forty. Most supermarket brands of vitamins use iron oxide as their "iron supplement." They are selling you *rust* in the name of nutrition. It can't really be absorbed by the body effectively.

Colloidal minerals (those provided by plant source) are 98 percent absorbable by the human body. The minerals and trace elements from plants are ten times more absorbable than metallic minerals because they are seven thousand times smaller than our red blood cells. They are negatively charged, so they have a natural attraction to the intestinal lining, which is positively charged.

We take colloidal minerals on a regular basis in my home because we know that every single day we fail to take a colloidal mineral supplement, we are increasing our risks of degenerative disease from mineral deficiencies.[20]

I've only scratched the surface of this important subject, so I encourage you to dig deeper into the subject of nutrition and the role vitamins, minerals and trace elements play in preventing disease and strengthening the human immune system. There are many other very important vitamins, minerals and trace elements that could not be covered simply because of space limitations. I believe I have covered the most important nutrients, and I hope I have sparked a desire to know more. If you have any questions about vitamin supplementation, please call my office at (800) 726-1834.

Now it is time to go on to the subject of fat and the role that different kinds of fat play in our health—or its demise.

PRACTICE PREVENTION
AND STAY HEALTHY
TODAY SO YOU WON'T
HAVE TO CURE AN
AVOIDABLE DISEASE
TOMORROW.

Six

TAKE YOUR DAILY
DOSE OF ESSENTIAL FAT!

ISN'T THIS A book about healthy living? How could any respectable nutrition authority tell someone, "Take your daily dose of essential fat"? The answer is simple: Not all fat is the same. In fact, it takes fat to burn fat! There are certain fats called *essential fatty acids* that help the body raise its metabolic levels or "turn up the heat" so fat reserves can be burned off. While your body can manufacture fat for storage from excess carbohydrates and dietary fat, it cannot manufacture these essential fatty acids. They must be supplied through what we eat or through dietary supplements.

When we get too much of the "bad" fat, our body stores it, greatly increasing our risk of heart and circulatory disease, cancer, diabetes and arthritis (and this is only the short list). All fat in your diet is a mixture of three different fatty acids.

The mix between saturated, monounsaturated and polyunsaturated fatty acids determines whether the fat is solid or liquid and how it will impact your health. Dietary fat that contains higher levels of saturated fatty acids tends to be solid at room temperature, and it has a higher melting point.

About 98 percent of the fat found in the foods we eat are mixed triglycerides. These complex molecules are made up of saturated, monounsaturated and polyunsaturated fats. Dr. John McDougall says, "If a test tube of blood is allowed to sit overnight on the counter, a layer of fat [triglycerides] will accumulate at the top by the next morning, as with chicken soup left overnight in the refrigerator. . . . High levels of triglycerides will sludge the blood, increase coagulation of the blood and cause insulin resistance."[1]

The most dangerous element among the triglycerides is saturated fat. Lard is nothing more than saturated pork fat, and butter is saturated dairy fat. The oils of certain plants such as cocoa butter (from the cacao bean), coconut oil and palm oil are also high in saturated fat and become solid at room temperature. These kinds of saturated fatty acids will stimulate your body's production of cholesterol and raise your "bad" cholesterol (LDL, or low-density lipoprotein) dramatically, increasing your risk for coronary heart disease.[2]

Unsaturated fatty acids come primarily from

plants. There are two types of unsaturated fatty acids: polyunsaturated fats, which are found in safflower, sunflower and corn oils, and monounsaturated fats, found in olive and canola oils.

WHAT ARE ESSENTIAL FATTY ACIDS?

WHEN WE SAY, "Take your daily dose of essential fat," we are talking about essential fatty acids. These are polyunsaturated fatty acids that are absolutely necessary for good health. Since the body is unable to manufacture them, we have to get them from the foods and supplements we eat. Children need essential fatty acids, including linoleic and linolenic acids, to ensure normal growth. Both children and adults need them to maintain healthy skin and to produce hormone-like substances crucial for regulating blood pressure and immune responses. These same unique fats also increase the body's ability to lubricate the joints.

Linoleic acid is an Omega-6 fatty acid found in plants, and linolenic acid is an Omega-3 fatty acid found in all fish and seafood, especially cold-water fish such as salmon, sardines and lake trout. Omega-6 fatty acids have been proven to have a cardio-protective dimension, and they are found in natural plant sources such as evening primrose and flaxseed oil.[3] Omega-3 fatty acids may help to prevent blood clots that lead to heart attack or stroke, and they may also help to prevent hardening of the arteries.[4]

Eighty years ago, about 40 percent of the fat in American diets was in the form of Omega-3 fatty acids, and about 60 percent was Omega-6 fatty acids. Now almost 90 percent of the fats we eat are saturated fats that are detrimental to our health, and some people don't get any of the essential Omega-3 and Omega-6 fatty acids in their diets.

The problem with fat is that our bodies were designed by our Creator to operate with very little of it. The foods we eat today—unlike the foods generally eaten by the human race in previous centuries—are very high in fat. We eat like kings, and we suffer and die of the same diseases that used to be unique to kings and other members of privileged classes. Kings were often known for their obesity and rich lifestyles, and they were often plagued by gout, arthritis and diabetes, to name a few diseases.[5]

An artery is a pipeline of life for the body. It is designed to transport blood—and the oxygen and nutrients it contains—to every part of the human body. Like any pipe, an artery can get clogged with deposits that aren't supposed to be there. I believe that is why God tells us, "You must never eat any fat or blood. This is a permanent law for you and all your descendants, wherever they may live" (Lev. 3:17). When God put together our plumbing,

He knew what would work and what would not work. Most of us mumble something about "being free from the law" and continue to eat large portions of our high-fat, marbled meats, pork and high-fat desserts because we think the thick texture of fat on our tongue makes the food taste better. Whom do we really think we are kidding? Do you really think that if you disagree with the Bible it will change the facts?

BAD THINGS HAPPEN WHEN THE CHOLESTEROL DAM BREAKS

WHEN ENOUGH OF this waxy material called *cholesterol* (specifically the "bad" cholesterol) builds up on an artery wall, it acts like a dam and closes off the openings to high traffic areas around the heart and brain. This causes your blood pressure to increase as your heart labors even harder to force blood through the clogged areas to get life-sustaining oxygen and food to your brain and heart muscles. This can cause chunks of this cholesterol dam to break off as blood clots.

Blood clots are dangerous, because they tend to be pushed toward smaller and smaller arteries until they can't go any further. Two vital areas of your body are very sensitive to anything that blocks off blood flow—even for a matter of seconds: your heart and your brain.

Most people think the heart gets plenty of oxygen and nutrients from the blood because it has all the blood in the body passing through it. The fact is that there is a special series of arteries to feed and oxygenate the muscle complex that we call the heart.

Red blood cells are approximately seven microns in diameter, and a small blood vessel measures about four microns in diameter.

The only way red blood cells can pass through these small blood vessels to feed heart muscle tissues is if they literally fold over. The tiny capillaries feeding the brain respond in the same way. A problem arises when you have a high-fat meal, because the fat-laden red blood cells have a tendency to stick together in a clump. That means they can't efficiently feed the heart through the smaller capillaries encircling your heart and brain—especially if you already have cholesterol build up or plaques on the walls of those blood vessels.

SIESTA TIME AT THE GREAT FAMILY FEAST

FORTY MINUTES AFTER the long-awaited high-fat meal on Thanksgiving Day, Easter or at the family reunion, everyone is lying on a couch taking a nap. They are not getting enough oxygen flowing to their brains, so they want to go sleep it off. In our infinite wisdom, many of us like to drink several cups of hot coffee after eating a high-fat meal. Now the combination of a high-fat meal followed by several doses of caffeine will really get that over-taxed, underfed and underoxygenated heart to pump hard.

This is a prescription for disaster just waiting to happen. This combination of bad habits explains why statistics demonstrate that so many heart attacks take place after a large meal.

If our great feasts were limited to three or four binges per year only, our overall health probably wouldn't be compromised. The problem isn't the occasional family feast; it is our daily fixation with rich food and with the fast-food establishments lined up along America's busiest boulevards. The menus offered by most fast-food restaurant chains major on saturated fats, because even most of their nonbeef foods are quick-fried in high-pressure commercial deep fryers.

One summer I took a rafting trip with some men who dragged me to McDonald's for breakfast. They all had sausage biscuits, while I thought to myself, *I can't believe the eating habits of these guys.* They were fine men, but their eating habits weren't so fine. The first three mornings on our trip, my friends headed for the nearest fast-food joint for breakfast. Finally, after three days of hearing me badger them about pork, they began to eat just biscuits, which was a little better. Most fast-food menus major on fat, sugar and salt. No wonder it tastes so good—but what is it doing to your arteries?

What About Daily "Fat Calories"?

During a nutrition conference I attended recently we were told that the U.S. Government recommends that Americans limit their fat intake to no more than 30 percent of the calories they consume each day. This high percentage figure is absolutely erroneous, unless the saturated fat is kept to less than 5 to 10 percent of the total, as far as I and most nutritionists are concerned. Perhaps some bureaucrats in a back room in Washington told one another, "Well, the average American is getting between 60 and 70 percent of their calories from fat. We can't make the standard so low that it is going to be unrealistic. They will become discouraged." In other words, I wonder if someone in the government arbitrarily set the "fat number" at 30 percent in order to make it more acceptable to the public.

Again, most of the nutritionists and researchers to whom I've talked agree with my opinion that our daily saturated-fat consumption should be no more than 5 to 10 percent of our total caloric intake from saturated fat—period. Dr. Dean

Ornish, a respected author, research scientist and specialist in internal medicine, noted in his book, *Eat More, Weigh Less,* that while human society and eating patterns change rapidly, the human body adapts to change very, very slowly. The high-fat diet we eat today is a relatively new and dangerous development in the history of man. He writes, "You are eating a diet that the human body has not had time to adapt to."[6] Dr. Ornish clearly explains why traditional "dieting" only makes us "fatter" in the long run:

> When you overeat, your fat cells grow larger. If you keep overeating, you begin forming new fat cells. You also gain weight. The size of your fat cells may decrease if you restrict food intake for a while, *but the number does not.* This helps explain why it becomes harder to lose weight each time you go through the yo-yo cycle of gaining and losing weight. When you first lose weight by restricting the *amount* of food you eat, you lose *both muscle and fat tissue.* But when you gain weight back, you regain proportionately *more fat than you lost* [italics mine].[7]

Believe it or not, you have to take in fat if you want to lose fat. I am not talking about consuming saturated fat, but about essential fatty acids. The problem is that if your body doesn't get enough essential fatty acids to help it burn your stored body fat, then it will begin to sense it isn't getting enough fat because food is scarce. That is when your pancreas begins excreting insulin with the command: "Store the fat! Hard times are coming."

WITH WHAT KIND OF OIL SHOULD WE COOK?

MAKE THE NECESSARY changes so you won't have to use much oil of any kind, because oil is pure fat no matter how saturated it is. It has been shown by the American Heart Association, the American Diabetes Association and the American Cancer Society, as we've already stated, that an increased incidence of the diseases against which those associations are battling has been directly linked to the increased incidence of fat in the American diet. Learn how to reduce fat from your system now. If you don't learn now, then you will have to learn later when your doctor or cardiologist tells you your triglycerides and cholesterol levels are sky high, and that you may need heart bypass surgery!

Practice prevention and stay healthy today so you won't have to cure an avoidable disease tomorrow. People are always asking me, "What type of oil should I use?" I tell them that the best type of oil— and the oil my wife and I use—is cold-pressed pure virgin olive oil. It is the best monounsaturated fat that I've ever found. In fact, sometimes it even gives people relief from some of their constipation problems. Another type of oil that is OK is canola oil. But frankly, all other types of oil on your supermarket shelf should not be used.

EXCESS FAT AND YOUR ACHING JOINTS

DID YOU KNOW that arthritis is one of the most common diseases directly linked to excessive fat in the diet? In 1950, there were ten million people in this country who were suffering from arthritis. In 1995, there were thirty-seven million people with this disease. Officials have predicted that if we follow current trends, *one out of every two* Americans who reach the age of sixty will have arthritis! Predictions estimate that we will have one million new cases of arthritis every single year.

Oddly enough, people suffering from arthritic conditions experience a 93 percent improvement in their symptoms when they take regular doses of cod liver oil. In the 1920s, Dr. Ralph Pemberton showed in his study that cod liver oil could eliminate pain and stiffness in the joints. Every joint is lubricated by synovial fluid, a mucous-like substance manufactured by an organ called the *bursae*. Dr. Pemberton found that people with arthritis who began taking cod liver oil would show a fifteen-fold improvement in the lubrication of the synovial fluid. People suffering from arthritis of the joints need that much improvement in their synovial fluid to increase their range of motion in the joints.

Early in 1999 I suffered a shoulder injury. The injury plagued me for four months. When I started using 1 tablespoon of cod liver oil three times a day with meals, my shoulder injury cleared up in just several weeks. Why does it seem it me that I always have to learn from personal experience?

Several years ago, I developed a serious case of "tennis elbow" that just wouldn't heal. Finally I realized that part of the problem was my limited fat intake—I needed to make sure that my body was getting the essential Omega-3 and Omega-6 fatty acids in my diet on a regular basis. As soon as I started supplementing my diet with flaxseed oil and evening primrose oil, my elbow immediately began to improve.

Two Fats You Can't Do Without

WE NEED TO make sure we supply our bodies with essential fatty acids that they are unable to manufacture or synthesize on their own. I recommend daily supplementation of your diet with flaxseed oil, evening primrose oil and cod liver oil on a regular basis (all of which are available in capsule form).

This is especially important for women because these essential fatty acids help restore and maintain the elasticity of the skin. I have seen people come in with premature wrinkling who began to correct their essential fatty-acid deficiencies with these oils. Their wrinkles started clearing up without any type of facial surgery or chemical phenol peel—all they did was simply to change the amount of fatty acids they put into their system.

Every morning after my wife and I work out, we have a protein shake to make sure we get maximum nutrients into our body (about 80 percent of your nutrient uptake after a workout occurs within two hours if you train regularly). When we fix that protein shake, we put either flaxseed oil in it or take some cod liver oil in capsule form. You won't taste it, but it will help facilitate the burning of fat in your body. It is one of the most efficient things that you can do to help to supply essential fatty acids. I recommend that you take three to four cod liver oil capsules with every meal. In addition to cod liver oil, you need to be taking evening primrose oil and flaxseed oil capsules every single day for healthy skin and complexion. (I know I am being redundant on this recommendation, but I feel it is that important!)

It is very important that you provide these essential fatty acids to your body while eliminating all excess saturated fat from your daily diet. Essential fatty acids cannot do their job alone. They play a role as part of a health-guarding team that includes wise food-consumption habits, natural vitamin and antioxidant supplementation, an abundance of pure water with dietary fiber and consistent exercise. If you're feeling a little confused about how to implement a healthy eating program, please call my office at 1-800-726-1834 for more information on my Eat, Drink and Be Healthy tape series and cookbook.

CONSISTENT EXERCISE
IS THE BEST WAY TO
KEEP YOUR ENERGY
LEVELS HIGH WHILE
IMPROVING THE
WAY YOU FEEL.

Seven

CHOOSE EXERCISE—
IT'S A DECISION YOU
CAN LIVE WITH

O NCE YOU PASS the physical age of twenty, you will lose 6 to 7 percent of your total muscle mass *every ten years* unless you are exercising on a regular basis! Regular exercise can literally keep you from "fading away" as you advance in age. Because overall body weight will tend to *go up,* or at best remain the same, most people don't realize that they continue to lose body muscle as they get older. Between the ages of twenty and seventy, you could lose approximately *30 percent* of your muscle mass due to tissue atrophy! The bad news is that you already know what replaces that muscle mass: fat.

But here is some very good news: This loss of muscle mass can be prevented or greatly reduced in most cases if you consistently use resistance training to exercise your muscles, eat wisely and drink plenty of pure water. This will keep your muscle cells healthy and well-supplied with glucose and other essential body fluids. Not only is consistent exercise the best way to avoid muscle loss in your senior years, but it also helps to keep your energy levels high while improving the way you feel.

Consistent exercise will also help keep your *weight* gain under control. Eighty percent of the calories or energy your body consumes is burned by your muscles. Yet exercise should always be accompanied by wise, thoughtful lifestyle habits. (Notice that I did not say a "diet.") Aging is a natural process for all living things, but there is no reason for us to accelerate the process through heart-clogging inactivity or food abuse at the dinner table.

When I discuss this issue of exercise in many of my public seminars, someone usually hits me with this question: "Ted, don't you know that the Bible says that 'bodily exercise profiteth little'?" (See 1 Timothy 4:8, KJV.)

The New Living Translation says this: "Physical exercise *has some value,* but spiritual exercise is much more important, for it promises a reward in both this life and the next" (1 Tim. 4:8, emphasis added). Five other Bible versions say much the same thing.

Paul was warning Timothy about religious leaders who expected others to meet the leaders' own private requirements before they could earn salvation and God's favor—things God never said or demanded. No matter how perfectly you develop your body or observe outward rules and regulations about what to wear or eat, you will still die some day. All your physical and mental efforts to reach perfection will fail to move you one inch closer to God or to His dwelling place in heaven!

Don't misuse Paul's warning about the limited value of exercise to save your soul as an excuse for physical negligence or a lazy lifestyle. Physical exercise was a normal part of everyday life in Bible times. Automobiles didn't exist in Paul's day, and people walked everywhere they went. Just the effort of living without labor-saving conveniences helped people maintain a reasonable degree of physical fitness. You aren't living under those conditions.

Paul's warning that "exercise profiteth little" rings very true in another sense for Americans: Exercise is a poor remedy for a lack of self-discipline at the dinner table. Considering the kinds of food we eat today, it is too easy to pile on the calories and very difficult to take them off. It gets even tougher after you reach the age of forty.

If you decide to take a brisk walk to "burn off that one-hundred-calorie tablespoon of butter you had with your evening meal," you will have to walk three miles to accomplish your goal! Wouldn't it be a little easier to "just say no" to that pat of butter?

Or would you want to run a full mile to burn off that pat of butter? You could also burn off that butter by cycling for five miles, swimming continuously for seven hundred yards, playing fifty minutes of highly competitive singles' tennis or by playing nonstop handball or racquetball for thirty minutes! Believe me, it's easier to pass on the butter. But if you are going to use butter, use it rather than margarine. I'll tell you why in a later chapter.

HORMONES AND METABOLISM:
THE MISSING PIECE OF THE PIE

MOST OF THE diet fads, and even the official government position of pushing a high-protein, high-carbohydrate, low-fat diet, are based on selected pieces of the nutritional puzzle rather than on the whole picture. Two of the most important missing pieces are the "basal metabolic rate" and two hormones that govern the way your body burns calories and stores fat.

No country on earth is more preoccupied with dietary fat than the United States, yet there is no nation on earth whose citizens are nearly as fat as Americans. Why? Year after year my office has been deluged with telephone calls from people wanting to know how they could lose weight and keep it off. Most of them admit to failing miserably with numerous diet plans.

When I was younger, I always tried to encourage these people to "stick with their diet plans." For me, gaining or losing weight had always been a matter of adding or eliminating a few foods from my diet, so I wrongly assumed that all these people needed was "more will power." Needless to say, some of the people who came to me suffering with a weight problem went away without improvement.

Then I reached the age of forty. For twenty years I had worked in the field of diet and nutrition while maintaining a disciplined personal exercise program. When I went on a tour, I would sometimes put on a few pounds and simply "work it off" after a week or two in the gym. After my fortieth year, I began to put on two to three pounds during extended trips. I could lose the first pound quickly, but the last two pounds stubbornly refused to leave me before I was off on another tour.

THE WEIGHT REMAINED DESPITE EXERCISE AND DIET

I WAS EXERCISING just as strenuously as before, but the extra weight clung to me like polyester pants filled with static electricity. What did I do? I took the commonly accepted advice of the scientific community and radically reduced my dietary fat intake.

I tend to be an "everything-or-nothing" type of person (as if you didn't already know that), so I consumed too little fat. My body couldn't produce enough essential fatty acids to nourish my skin, which became dry and flaky (a process we discussed in the previous chapter on our body's need for essential fatty acids). Even with this extremism, the weight still fought me. I began to have a new and personal understanding of the mental anguish experienced by people battling chronic weight problems.

I spent weeks pondering the current literature on diet and human biochemical relationships between diet and weight gain. The question kept coming to my mind, *Is there something wrong with my body or my metabolism?* Finally it occurred to me: The problem was *hormonal.*

As my age increased, the various hormonal levels in my body had changed. Hormones regulate all of the key nutritional processes of the body, including blood sugar levels and fat storage. When this delicate balance is altered, things begin to change quickly. In my case, my hormonal balance changed with age and made it much more difficult for me to lose body fat. (Experts now call it male menopause.)

My scientific search for understanding of my own weight problem has become a key to helping hundreds of thousands of other people control their weight and reclaim the energy they've lost. Your hormones regulate bodily functions, and your "basal metabolic rate" helps regulate your hormones. Therefore, the real secret to maintaining muscle mass and losing unhealthy body fat is learning how to increase your basal metabolic rate.

Most people are familiar with the hormones testosterone and estrogen (the most prominent sexual hormones for men and women respectively). The body also produces other hormones for very specific tasks or functions. The thyroid hormone regulates the overall metabolism rate of the body. Antidiuretic hormones regulate the water balance of the body through the kidneys, and insulin and glucagon regulate the metabolism of food (specifically glucose) and the production and burning of fat. Insulin and glucagon are the hormones responsible for fat gain and the difficulty we have in losing it.

This little fact accounts for one of the biggest national health policy failures in recent years. In the 1980s, scientists began to warn us about the hazards of consuming too much dietary fat. They cursed red meat, egg yolks and poultry skins while touting the virtues of a high-carbohydrate, low-fat diet. They assured us that weight loss would be instantaneous and pain free. Manufacturers got into the act and began producing new low-fat and fat-free products aimed at satisfying the public's new demand for these so-called healthy products. The scientists were sincere, but we have now discovered that they were also very wrong.

After months of research about my "battle with the bulge," I realized that the high-carbohydrate, low-fat diet I was on *actually made matters worse!* How could that be? Didn't the American Medical Association announce that all Americans should eat a high-carbohydrate, low-fat diet to avoid the risks of heart disease and cancer (not to mention obesity)? The truth is that the high-carbohydrate, low-fat diets promoted by current literature as the salvation of overweight Americans has had devastating effects on our health *as far as weight is concerned.*

Fifteen years have passed since the scientific revelation about the miracle high-carbohydrate, low-fat diet. Therefore, it seems logical to assume that many Americans have successfully shed most of their unwanted pounds. After all, we are consuming much less fat and many more carbohydrates, *so we should be thinner, right?* Wrong.

How Do We Eat Less and Gain More?

According to the National Center for Health Statistics in the Centers for Disease Control and Prevention, *prior* to the revelation of the high-carbohydrate, low-fat diet, *about 25 percent of the*

American population was so overweight that they were classified as obese.

Only *eleven years* after the high-carbohydrate, low-fat diet campaign was launched, the number of Americans classified as obese had risen to *32 percent!* Government statistics actually indicate that every man, woman and child in the United States have gained an average of ten pounds in less than a decade! We supposedly adopted a healthier way of eating, and we've made jazzercise and aerobics a national pastime. Still, the government says we are consuming dramatically less fat while becoming dramatically fatter! Why?

MEET YOUR HORMONAL TWINS: THE FAT MASTERS

AS I MENTIONED before, the problem is *hormonal* (even if most of us are *not* teenagers), and the specific hormonal twins at the core of the problem are *insulin* and *glucagon.* Both are manufactured and released into the blood stream by the pancreas. Exercise and diet together play a key role in maintaining their proper balance in the body.

Insulin is secreted into the system after we eat as a response to rising levels of sugars in the blood stream, and for this reason it is the hormone associated with diabetes. When we consume a meal, the food we eat is broken down into protein, fat and carbohydrates. When carbohydrates are digested, they are broken down further into glucose, or sugar—the body's main fuel source. It is glucose that travels through the blood system bringing nourishment to all the cells of the body.

So far, all this information seems to support the high-carbohydrate diet claims. But there is another problem to consider, one that brings hormones right back into the picture: *Glucose cannot enter a cell directly on its own.*

The internal environment of our cells is highly regulated, and large molecules such as glucose are kept out by dense cell walls that protect the inner parts of the cell. Insulin works much like a key to unlock cellular gateways so that glucose can enter and bring nourishment. (Actually, insulin is more like a "boot" that forces glucose into cells, as we shall see later.)

Insulin is also responsible for reducing levels of glucose in the blood stream after the consumption of sugary meals. This is why some people with diabetes must receive daily injections of insulin to control their blood sugar levels. Under normal circumstances, when we eat an extra serving of dessert with ice cream, our blood sugar can rise to dangerously high levels in a matter of minutes. The pancreas secretes insulin to lower these sugar levels immediately by forcing glucose into our body cells.

The key link between weight gain, exercise and

insulin is found in the next function of this important hormone: Insulin is also a storage hormone that causes the body to store fuel for later use. "Storage" is where the problem begins for the overweight individual.

Remember that glucose is the main fuel source for the body, and it is the *only* fuel source for the brain. Despite the crucial importance of glucose as its primary fuel source, the body has a very limited capacity to store glucose in its purest forms. The purest form of instantly available "stored" glucose is *glycogen,* a hormone that is the "twin sister" of insulin. This hormone, which is manufactured by the pancreas, is found almost exclusively in the liver and muscle tissues.

Only about 400 grams (sixteen hundred calories) of glucose can be stored in the body at any one time. The liver holds about 100 grams, and muscles hold 300 grams.

Let me put this in perspective for you. Sixteen hundred calories isn't a lot of extra fuel. If you stopped eating for some reason, this reserve of sixteen hundred calories could become depleted after merely thirty to sixty minutes of intense exercise. At first glance, it seems simple for the body to replenish such a small "gas tank," and that is correct. You can fill up that sixteen-hundred-calorie tank with only one high-carbohydrate meal after your exercise time.

WHERE DOES ALL THAT EXTRA "FUEL" GO?

THE PROBLEM IS that very few people really "empty" their tank of glucose, so they are loading up with *excess* carbohydrates every time they eat a meal. This is where insulin becomes a serious problem. As you recall, the digestive system always converts carbohydrates into glucose, or sugar, that is absorbed into the blood stream. This triggers the instant release of insulin into the bloodstream.

Once insulin has done its job of forcing glucose into the body's cells, the glucose must commit to one of three things:

1. It can be used for energy immediately.
2. It can be stored as glycogen in the liver or muscle tissues (but only 400 grams may be stored at any one time).
3. It can be (*and usually is*) stored as fat.

The short version of this story is that when your glycogen "gas tank" is full, glucose has no choice but to be turned into fat. So what really happens to all those calories you consume when you eat a high-carbohydrate meal? You already know. If they are not burned or used to replace your standard 400-gram glycogen reserve, then your body will turn those calories into fat—even if you have carefully reduced your intake of dietary fat!

Two Biochemical Facts Everyone Should Know

1. *Once glucose has been converted to fat, it can* never *be converted back to glucose.* Fat is a structure that has no ability to convert to sugar or even to muscle. The only way to get rid of fat is to burn it off through—you've guessed it—*consistent aerobic and resistance exercise.*

2. *Protein, however, can be converted to glucose.* This can be seen in the way our bodies respond to starvation. Since glucose is needed as fuel for the brain, any time the human body is deprived of food (for instance, through a fad diet), it becomes a super-efficient scavenger. It begins to raid existing body tissues for *stored protein* (i.e., muscle tissues) to convert into glucose. This is the body's way of preserving vital brain tissues by providing its own nourishment when it is deprived of food.

This second biochemical reaction—the ability to convert protein into glucose—is important to understanding how the body can best convert fuels and *lose fat without losing muscle.*

How does all this relate to exercise and the high-carbohydrate, low-fat diet? The scientists were right in the 1980s when they told us that the body was designed to get its fuel primarily from carbohydrates. They simply went too far when they told us to *overdose* on them through a high-carbohydrate diet. They were also right to warn us about the dangers of a high-fat diet, but they were wrong to put a curse on *all fats* (including essential fatty acids).

The high-carbohydrate, low-fat diet also overlooked the crucial relationship of insulin to weight gain and the function of excess carbohydrates as a natural trigger to higher levels of insulin secretion. Insulin's job is to lower sugar levels in the blood and to store the extra. Biochemically, the insulin hormone does its job as a storage hormone by effectively *blocking the body's ability to break down fat and burn it off.*

The pancreas responds to the excessive carbohydrates in the typical American meal by secreting insulin, which keeps us from burning off the excess body fat we already have. And it converts the carbohydrates we eat into even more body fat!

Where Is the Hero in This Picture?

Now if insulin is the villain in the battle of the bulge, there must be a hero hormone to come to our rescue, right? There is, and its name is *glucagon.* It comes from the same place as its rival, insulin. Glucagon is secreted by the pancreas to *raise blood glucose levels* by freeing stored glucose from the muscle tissues and the liver. It also acts to stimulate the breakdown of fat energy, thereby putting a halt to fat storage.

It is clear that if we want to lose excess fat and maintain maximum energy levels, we must increase levels of glucagon while decreasing levels of insulin. How? Exercise and reduced high-glycemic carbohydrate meals are the only ways I know. Reduced carbohydrate meals prevent large quantities of insulin from being produced in the first place, while protein actually stimulates glucagon production. Exercise also stimulates glucagon production, perhaps better than a low-carbohydrate meal.

When I jumped on the high-carbohydrate, low-fat diet bandwagon, hoping to lose my extra three pounds, I didn't realize that I was sending a major action message to my pancreas with every meal. It responded to the high levels of glucose-producing carbohydrates by releasing large amounts of insulin into my bloodstream. This forced the overdose of glucose into my body cells. Again, there were only three places for all of that *excess* glucose to go. Some of it was burned as energy during my work-outs in the gym, but I could only burn so much at one time. Some of it could be stored as glycogen to replenish my 400-gram "gas tank." Most of it, however, was converted to fat for storage. I already had the exercise component of a healthy lifestyle in place, so when I reduced the amount of carbohydrates in my meals, my excess pounds came off and stayed off.

The only real way for your body to burn fat while saving muscle is to cause the body to reverse its production of storage hormones (insulin) and to stimulate the body's ability to produce fat-burning hormones (glucagon). The sensibility of this concept is obvious; however, it is also largely ignored by the majority of dietitians and nutritionists in this country.

We need to develop sensible dietary patterns that limit the ability of insulin to control our waistline. All it takes is for us to stop giving our bodies the foods that cause insulin to be produced in the first place. The only way to limit insulin production is to limit high-glycemic carbohydrate consumption. I know this sounds like nutritional heresy, but it is the "biochemical, hormonal gospel!" The best way to do this is to use a food glycemic index chart that tells you which foods to avoid. This is part of my Forever Fit tape series—a wise investment for everyone fighting the battle of the bulge.

A new lifestyle of eating must be established that will include "low-glycemic carbohydrates."

Researchers have carefully classified various foods according to the amount of blood sugar they produce in the blood stream over a three-hour period.[1] Not all carbohydrates produce extreme insulin reactions, and the "low-glycemic index" carbohydrates may be eaten at will and in virtually any quantity you desire. They include most fresh vegetables and some fruits. The "mean" or center reference point for the Glycemic Index is flour and wheat products such as whole wheat and white bread, which have an index of 100. Any food with a Glycemic Index of 70 and above is considered a high-glycemic index food, an insulin promoter and a glucagon inhibitor.[2]

Processed grains, including cereals, cakes, white rice and refined flour, must be considered luxuries and eaten conservatively. They cannot be the mainstay of your diet as they have been in the past. Continue to eat plenty of lean proteins with lots of vegetables and fresh fruits. An exercise program is a must, along with pure water and vitamin supplements.

THREE KINDS OF EXERCISE *YOU NEED* EVERY DAY

YOU ARE PROBABLY sitting as you read these words, and that is OK. But if you spend most of your time sitting, that is not healthy. If you are serious about getting maximum energy every day, if you really want to live a life free of excess weight and the health problems associated with it, then your weekly routine should include at least three different types of exercise.

Cardiovascular exercise

You should be doing some kind of continuous *cardiovascular exercise* for twenty to thirty minutes at least three to five times a week. (Before beginning any exercise program, check with your medical doctor.) By cardiovascular exercise, I am referring to physical exertion that puts a healthy load on the heart, the lungs and the complex network of blood vessels, veins and capillaries in your body. Blood vessels and the heart are just like your muscles—they grow stronger with regular use and healthy exercise.

If possible, this should be done first thing in the morning before any calories are drunk or eaten. By training on an empty stomach, the body will release glucagon from the pancreas to facilitate the burning of fat for fuel. I have personally lowered my own body fat levels by 5 percent this past year by implementing this approach to training.

No, you don't have to go outside and run three miles a day, but you should do something like walking, swimming, cycling, participating in a low-impact aerobics class or putting in some time on a treadmill. (I prefer low-impact cardiovascular exercises that are easy on the joints and ligaments—particularly for people who are over the age of forty. It is also strongly recommended that you check with your health practitioner before beginning any kind of exercise or diet modification program.)

The goal of cardiovascular exercise is to *accelerate the heart rate for a sustained period of time and to burn body fat if needed.* Now if you are over forty, don't tell yourself, "Well, I am going to start running thirty minutes every day now for the next five years." Chances are that you may not make it. After the first day they may be wheeling you into the ambulance and on to the hospital. Everyone has to acknowledge the changes that come to the body as the years add on. Also remember you may not have had any exercise since high school—so take it easy. You have the rest of your life to get in shape. Regardless of your age, cardiovascular exercise is absolutely important for proper health. If all you can do is walk around the block every night, then do it. If it's winter time and too cold to walk, then get yourself a treadmill or an elliptical runner such as a Precor.

Flexibility training

Another very important aspect of any daily fitness program is *flexibility training.* (We used to call it "stretching.") This kind of training can prevent much of the immobility associated with aging, and it prevents the kind of joint and ligament problems that many people suffer when they begin their workouts without properly warming up their body tissues.

Remember when Tim Conway used to do the comedy sketch of a little old man taking baby steps? Well, that can really happen if you don't stretch on a regular basis. Since my back surgery in 1988, I've implemented a daily stretching regime, and it has made a huge difference in my flexibility.

If you haven't done any flexibility training in a while, don't go overboard. You can quickly injure yourself by trying to force your joints, ligaments and muscles to do things they aren't used to doing. If you can bend over and touch your knees but no further, then work with that. Don't force yourself to go past where you can go, and never ever bounce. You will usually find that over time, your body will increase its flexibility, but take it easy. There are many books written on the topic—check out your local bookstore.

Strength training

You need to devote at least thirty to forty-five minutes to *strength training* three times a week. This is true regardless of your age. An interesting study was conducted with a group of people in a nursing home who were confined to wheelchairs.

Several of these patients started a consistent strength-training program and were able to regain enough of their muscle mass to leave their wheelchairs. They began to enjoy light sports such as walking, golf and softball! Isn't it amazing to see what our bodies can do when we just give them the proper exercise?

Is Your Twitch Slow or Fast?

STRENGTH TRAINING NECESSARILY involves muscles. Our bodies have "slow-twitch" muscles and "fast-twitch" muscles, as well as a type of muscle that is a combination of both. Each type of muscle fiber needs a different kind of exercise. For instance, fast-twitch muscle fibers are the explosive fibers. They are designed to effectively handle very heavy weights, and they can be built up to phenomenal size and bulk. When they are involved in intense work or strain, they produce a by-product of protein synthesis called lactic acid, characterized by a distinct burning sensation. This is what athlete and bodybuilders mean when they talk about weight-lifting exercises that cause muscles to "burn."

Do not ignore your body's signals. If you get a twinge of pain from a *joint* or *ligament,* pay attention to it, and stop doing whatever triggered the pain. The same is true if you think you may have strained a muscle. When I was younger, I did some strength-training exercises that weren't good for my spine and joints. In time I had to undergo back surgery that put me flat on my back for five weeks. It took me almost a year to regain my full strength. Don't ignore your body's built-in warning system.

Slow-twitch muscle fibers lack the explosive power of fast-twitch muscles, but they are built for the "long haul." These are the kinds of muscles used for long-distance endurance running. Everyone's body has both kinds of muscles, but there is a difference between the distribution of these muscles in each body. This explains why some men have the explosive power in their legs needed to run the Olympic one-hundred-yard dash or play tackle on a football team. Those same men would have difficulty keeping up with another person on a twenty-mile run. Why? Their bodies contain different concentrations of fast- and slow-twitch muscle fibers. We need to keep this in mind when we begin our strength training.

Never compare yourself to someone else. You are unique, so you need to develop a strength-training program that is custom-tailored to your body type, physiology and personal health goals. This is best done with the assistance of a knowledgeable exercise physiologist or personal trainer.[3]

HOW DID HE DO THAT?

DON'T BE DISCOURAGED if you don't work out with the same amount of weight or repetitions as someone else. What really matters is that you consistently exercise the body God gave you. I took a trip down memory lane to my college days recently when I saw a friend of mine with whom I used to work out. In those days I was frustrated, because no matter how hard I tried, I could only bench-press three hundred forty pounds. My friend Arnie would come into the gym twice a week, and he would *warm up* with three hundred forty pounds.

When I saw Arnie in the gym recently, he was still working out with three hundred fifty to four hundred pounds on the bench press. Over the years I had learned a lot about muscle mechanics. A friend of mine who is a college professor in sports physiology taught me about strength potential and joint angles. He told me that one of the key areas that is first checked out for a potential Olympic power lifter is where the elbow breaks when placed beside the head. So this time I asked Arnie to lift up his arm to see how high his elbow went above or below his head. When I saw that Arnie's elbow broke exactly even with his ear, it clicked! I thought, *Well, no wonder. I have spider arms compared to him—my elbow extends far beyond the top of my head.*

I had been foolishly comparing myself to Arnie in college, when the difference between us was really a matter of mathematical angles and leverage. Remember there are people who, because of their body composition and joint placement, will be stronger than you. My current workout partner is Van Green, a former defensive back for the Cleveland Browns. The man is in phenomenal shape. The other day I asked him how many pullups he could do. He casually strolled over to the pullup bar and did twenty-five perfect repetitions. He is an incredible world-class athlete, eats correctly, takes supplements, has a low percentage of body fat, is a minister of the gospel—and is forty-eight years old! I'm blessed to have such a motivator and mentor as a friend and training partner.

Don't confuse muscle weight with fat weight. Many times people don't lose much weight when they start to work out since muscle tissue is denser and heavier than body fat. You start gaining muscle weight at the same time that you start burning body fat, which explains why the weight scales don't seem to have moved despite all your physical effort. I urge my clients to limit themselves to one trip per week to the scales at the most. If you want to measure anything, measure body fat loss.

THE ORDERLY WAYS OF FAT

THE HUMAN BODY likes to store its excess fat in an orderly way, proceeding in order from the abdominal area to the deep tissue surrounding the abdominal area, followed by superficial areas around the body, then the buttocks, and lastly, the thighs and arms. When you start to lose excess weight, it will go off in the *same order.*

Don't believe all the ads you see and hear. There is no such thing as "spot reduction" through exercise, creams, diet supplements or any other miracle cure. The only way to "spot reduce" body fat is through an invasive medical procedure such as liposuction, which I only recommend as a last resort. However, if you do decide to have liposuction, make sure you use a board-certified plastic surgeon. I have seen disasterous results from liposuction done by doctors who have taken weekend classes and claim to be "trained." In fact, I know of one such weekend "trainee" who actually performed liposuction on a patient who had not been properly sedated. What a nightmare! What you *can* do is reduce overall body fat, which has countless benefits for your short- and long-term health.

If you really need to lose some weight, you need to make sure you lose fat and *not* lean muscle weight. The popular fad diets tend to produce short-term results by temporarily pulling water weight from your body by tricking your body into extracting nutrients from your muscle tissues in a starvation mode or through "metabolic weight loss" programs that skip exercise in favor of prescribed diet pills, thyroid medicine or sedatives. As we've already seen, you can lose body fat safely and permanently by modifying your eating patterns to pick up your basal metabolic rate combined with consistent exercise and the thoughtful use of vitamin supplements (which we covered in chapter five).

There are several other tips that you need to know about weight loss "magic pills." Don't use adrenal stimulation like mahuang and ephedrine to lose weight. Most of the herbal formulas are loaded with these products. These types of products can have serious side effects to the central nervous system and the cardiovascular system.

Let me tell you right up front that there are some days when I really don't want to go to the gym. I do it anyway for several reasons: First, I have kept at it long enough for daily exercise to become a habit. That is why I urge you to do the same. Don't commit to a trial run; commit to a new lifestyle with the fabulous payoff of better health, lower body fat, better appearance and higher energy levels. Second, I know in my heart of hearts that it is the right thing to do. It is the important thing to do. It is a life choice that I made a long time ago, and it's a decision that both you and I can live with.

For more information on my men's and women's exercise videos or my Forever Fit at 20, 30, 40 & Beyond series, please call my office at (800) 726-1834.

STRESS IS THE MOST WIDESPREAD MEDICAL PROBLEM IN AMERICA TODAY.

Eight

MANAGE STRESS
AND MAINTAIN YOUR BODY

A LOT OF PEOPLE are rushing in their workplace or career toward an early death in the name of "success and achievement." Forget it. It is not worth it. The artificially sustained energy levels (or should I say adrenaline levels?) and stress from this kind of self-made rat race will kill you long before your time.

Stress is one of the biggest problems in this country today. It can disrupt the human digestive system and inhibit the body's ability to absorb vital nutrients and replenish damaged or worn-out tissues. Excessive stress can be named as a causative factor or as an aggravating factor in nearly every disease and affliction known to man.

There are at least two categories of stress: the stress that we create ourselves through unreasonable internal expectations, and the stress brought into our lives by outside forces, individuals and circumstances. You have power over the stress that you have created. Begin by making sure your goals do not take precedence over your family priorities or your personal health. If you lose your job through layoffs or a plant closing, you can find another one. If you lose your health, you may never work again—if you survive at all.

WHAT CAN WE DO ABOUT STRESS?

WHAT IS THE solution? Begin by listening to your body's warning signals. If you are too tired to go out and do something tonight, then just stay at home and relax. Doesn't that make sense? Never eat in front of the TV. How stress-free will your stomach be if you eat your healthy, high-fiber, reduced-fat meal in front of a thirty-two-inch box showing nonstop murders, mayhem, arguments, violence, betrayal and physical and verbal abuse? (I am still talking about the evening news. I haven't even begun to describe the prime-time shows! They are stress carefully packaged in colorful bite-sized "sound bites" with commercials on both ends.) My wife and I very rarely watch television because of the stressful and incredibly negative things that continually flash across the screen. (If you do watch TV, always remember to mute all commercials.) The hectic pace of the images alone is enough to trigger the "fight-or-flight" reflex of the adrenal system.

Our bodies and spirits were simply not designed by God to hear all the negative news from around the world. Let's face it—most of us have enough stress simply trying to deal with the reality of our jobs and families. We don't need the continual barrage of news about school shootings, bombings, natural disasters and global conflicts. I mean enough is enough. I often tell my wife that CNN stands for "constant negative news."

LEARN HOW TO RELAX

ONE OF THE most important keys to living with maximum energy in your life is the ability to truly relax. I am a classic "Type A" individual who tends to be "driven" to achieve and accomplish preset goals. That means I can easily become my own worst enemy in the area of relaxation. I've learned personally and professionally through years of research that you can only relax by learning how to control your thoughts and emotions.

Stress is the most widespread medical problem in America today. It has literally been linked to every major disease that plagues mankind. Your best defense against the ravages of excess stress begins with the "one-two" combination of a consistent exercise program and a low-fat, high-fiber diet, which we have already covered. There is more that you can do as well: You can learn how to handle stressful situations wisely, and you can learn how truly to relax when you are away from those situations.

No one is immune from stress. Stress is the body's nonspecific response to any demands placed upon it, whether those demands are pleasant or not.

You can have good stress, or you can have bad stress. It doesn't matter because *all stress* affects the body—and the digestive system in particular—in the same way.

HOW TO ENJOY PARADISE IN GRIDLOCK

ADVERSE CONDITIONS CAN raise your stress levels almost instantly. Anyone who has driven a car or a forty-foot motor coach in rush-hour traffic knows what I am talking about. I remember one time I was caught in the middle of a gridlocked super-highway in our motor coach when I suddenly realized how stressful I felt. Finally I said, "OK, Lord, I just need to kick back and relax." I maneuvered our "ship on wheels" into the right-hand lane with everybody else and settled in at a breathtaking two miles an hour. *Forget it,* I thought. *It doesn't matter. I'll get to where I'm going—just a little slower—but with a lot less stress and danger.*

I put on some good music and just relaxed. Sometimes I even found myself so relaxed that I slowed down traffic a little more. (Sorry, all of you uptight types.) I set the cruise control at a slow speed and told myself, "I will chop through the traffic a foot at a time, and sooner or later I will get through it." One key to handling stress is not to let people or circumstances around you control you.

When you drive a large motor coach, there are times when you just have to pull out if you ever hope to enter a traffic lane or make a turn. It is amazing how many people tell me with their upraised fingers of salutation that I am "number one"! (Yes, that is my sanitized, reframed version of what they are saying.) When they do, I just turn to my lovely wife and say, "Look, Sharon, those people must love us. They think I am number one. Isn't that great?" Then I wave at them. That makes them think that they have accidentally "saluted" someone they know, and most of the time it really embarrasses them. Usually these "fans" end up waving back with a look that says, "Oh, no." It is a great way of reducing the stress in a potentially difficult situation. I mean, why am I going to lower myself to that type of nonverbal stressful conversation?

One day I was driving my trusty coach through gridlocked traffic in Boston, trying to find my way to an unfamiliar location. (I wish people would have a little more patience with people from other cities and regions—it isn't easy navigating through busy traffic as a visitor in a large city.) There seems to be an unwritten law of physics that says visitors must always end up in the wrong traffic lane in gridlocked traffic, and I was obediently occupying forty feet in the wrong lane. The only way out of the situation was to speed up and merge into the next lane. Naturally, I had to move in front of another man, but I made sure there were four or five car lengths between us. Evidently it wasn't enough.

This man pulled up beside me, rolled down his window and started screaming at me. He went absolutely berserk. So I rolled down my window and politely said, "Pardon me? I can't hear you. Could you please help me? I am lost, and I need some directions."

The man's whole countenance changed. He said, "Well, I didn't mean to get upset."

I smiled and said, "That's OK; it didn't hurt me. I didn't hear you. The point is that you really need to calm down a little bit."

He looked at me with a sheepish smile and said, "You know, you're right." Remember: Don't let yourself be affected by people you don't even know.

The only people who can really get me upset are the people I really love and care about, and that is if they intentionally do something wrong. Too many of us live under the weight of stress our whole lives, worried about what some stranger is going to think because our hair is not perfect or because we didn't shave. Listen, nobody really cares.

FORGET THE IMAGINARY PREDATORS

WHEN YOU PUT yourself under stress, it burns up much of your energy, and it tells your body to release incredibly powerful adrenaline and other hormones into your body. When your body clicks into the "fight-or-flight" mode, you have activated the protective state your Creator gave you to run from predators or fight off attackers. When you just sit and fume—or eat, fume and drop into a fitful sleep—those hormones don't help you. They increase your heart rate dramatically, raise your blood pressure and tense your muscles, causing tremendous damage to your body over the long run. You have spent a life fighting with "imaginary predators" that don't even exist—with no aerobic benefit to show for it.

Chronically tense muscles result in numerous psychosomatic disorders, headaches, muscle spasms and other unpleasant physical symptoms. When you are dealing with rush-hour traffic, make sure that your mouth is opened a little so your jaws won't clench. Make sure you are not gripping the steering wheel too tightly—unless you are competing in a Grand Prix race where you have to hold onto the steering wheel tightly to make tight turns. Don't drive like that around the country or in city traffic—you might not make it.

Identify what is stressful so you can cope with it. Talk to someone about it, and plan ahead to avoid or minimize the stress if possible. Many people feel stressful because it is so difficult to get to work on time. Manage that stress by leaving for work ten minutes earlier—you probably won't have any stress at all. Don't wait until the last possible second hoping the traffic will be perfect so you can get there on time. It won't be, and you won't be on time either.

No, Thank You—Keep Your Snakes

Tackle the problems one by one as you approach them. Have a positive attitude. How you perceive and think about a problem makes all the difference. Positive attitudes may not alleviate all your problems, but it is always better to approach problems with a positive attitude than with a negative one. Sometimes you will meet people who are interested in talking only about how bad things are all the time. I don't have the time or patience for that. If someone brought a basket of angry, deadly poisonous pit vipers to your front door and said, "This is Acme Delivery Service. Will you sign for this package?", you would simply tell them, "Nope, we don't want them. You can keep those snakes. Send them back where they came from." Do the same when an overload of stress presents itself to you—send it back; don't internalize it.

One of the lesser-known casualties of the Industrial Revolution and our "urban-dweller" mind-set is the amount of time we spend outside. The Creator designed our bodies to thrive in an environment with plenty of fresh air and sunshine. The largest organ in your body is your skin. This highly developed organ is designed to manufacture vitamin D when it is exposed to daylight. It also helps to provide your body tissues with oxygen and moisture drawn from the air. That is why your body has such a sense of refreshment when you step outside into a gentle summer breeze or crisp fall wind, or when you feel the warmth of the sun on your face. That sense of well-being is your body's instinctive response to its natural environment.

We were not designed to live in real or artificial caves that are lit by artificial light and ventilated by stagnant bacterial-contaminated, closed-system, air-handling systems. One of the best ways to handle stress when it gets out of hand is to step away from your desk or home and take a walk outside. It will improve your mental well-being and give you a sense of inner peace.

FIVE WAYS TO MANAGE YOUR THOUGHTS

MY WIFE AND I spend a lot of time traveling the nation on an ongoing basis to teach people how to achieve top performance on the job and in their lives. We teach them how to provide proper nutrition for their bodies, and we teach them several ways to manage their thought life. Use these principles in your own life:

1. Focus your thoughts and attitudes.
Remember, all the yesterdays can never outweigh today. Yesterday is gone forever— today and tomorrow are the rest of your life. There is nothing that you can do to retrieve yesterday. We all have the same amount of hours in our days and the same number of days per week. Learn to slow down and think about today. Take control of your thought processes and decide where you will focus your mind. Success begins with the art of taking life one day at a time. Sure, you can make plans, but you will pursue those plans one day at a time. Jesus told us, "So don't worry about tomorrow, for tomorrow will bring its own worries. Today's trouble is enough for today" (Matt. 6:34).

2. Reframe negative situations into positive ones.
Learn how to be a "good-finder." If you don't do as well as you had hoped while trying to imple-

ment the things you've learned in this book, simply say, "I didn't do exactly what I was supposed to do today, but I have twenty-nine more days to do well. I'm still going to achieve my goal."

Avoid thinking, *I will never reach that goal; I just can't do it.* As long as you still have breath in your lungs and life in your spirit, you have everything you need to succeed. Just keep moving toward your goal *one day at a time.*

3. Eliminate any words that put you in a negative state.

I removed several words from my daily vocabulary because they always put me in a negative state. I try never to use the word *hate* any more. It is a negative word that doesn't do anything but conjure up negative images in your mind that produce negative chemical and physical reactions in your body and nervous system. It is a word that produces death instead of life, so it has been removed from my daily vocabulary, along with words like *stupid, idiot* and *shut up.*

You may be thinking, *Ted, why in the world are you talking about this? What does it have to do with an "energy advantage"?* Eliminating negative words from our vocabulary has *everything* to do with success in life and with our daily energy levels. The mental arena, particularly the subconscious mind, plays a vital role in how well you perform from day to day—and for the rest of your life.

Learn how to reframe your words. If you don't like something your spouse or child does, say, "Honey, you do so well most of the time. In fact, it is wonderful to see how well you do most of the time. But do you think we could work on this one area a little bit more? To be honest, it kind of bothers me a little bit, and I don't want anything to come between us."

4. You bring about what you speak about.

When I earned my degree in psychology at Florida State, I learned that the average person has about fifty thousand thoughts a day pass through his or her mind. Those thoughts will either build us up or tear us down. Only a few of those thoughts will actually be expressed through the words we speak. Here is my point: We bring about what we speak about. The Bible says, "For as [a person] thinks within himself, so he is" (Prov. 23:7, NAS).

One of the most important things that I can tell you is this: If you constantly tell yourself, "This is too hard. I can't do it. I'm destined to fail," then your mind will not disappoint you. Your mind will find a way to make your words become a self-fulfilling prophecy.

I knew a man who launched a very successful home-based business. He did very well until he reached the point where he made more money than he had ever expected to make. All of a sudden he began to do things that can only be described as "self-sabotage." He did everything he possibly could over a two-month period to reduce his income back to the level he had before he became successful. His self-defeating thought life short-circuited his potential for success.

Let me give you another example. I had a friend in high school who was extremely negative—just as I was at that time. After undergraduate studies, he went on to law school, and I went to graduate school at Florida State University. While in graduate school, I became a Christian. My whole life changed, and I began to work on becoming more positive about life.

When I shared my newfound hope with my friend in law school, he ridiculed me, sending me a super-negative, nasty letter telling me not to contact him again.

Several years later while driving drunk, he had an accident and killed a young passenger in his car. He received a three-year mandatory prison sentence and lost his law license. Today he is one of the most negative, bitter, disliked men in his community.

I believe his whole life has turned out horribly because his thought life forced him—and I literally mean *forced* him—to choose poorly.

Learn to choose wisely and positively. Recognize the crossroads of choice—it may only come once—and make the choice that will position you for success.

Success can sometimes trigger an invisible "thermostat" on the wall of our minds. If we set the thermostat for "eighty degrees of success," but our forward progress in life takes us past our preset "eighty degree" success limit, the subconscious mind can kick in to drop us back down to a preset comfort level. It seems irrational, but once we reach a level of success or achievement that is incongruent (or inconsistent) with what we believe we deserve, then our mind may subconsciously try to find a way to change it. Why? Because deep inside we believe we can't stay at such an uncomfortable level. This kind of thing happens when we branch out into new business ventures or romantic relationships. It can happen when we receive corporate promotions or commit ourselves to a healthier lifestyle of revised eating patterns and a physical exercise regimen.

5. As my friend Zig Ziglar always says, "Avoid spending too much time with people who 'brighten up a room by leaving it.'"

Have you noticed that when you ask most people how they are doing, they will give you a thirty-minute "organ recital" on how badly they feel and how badly things are going? Some people have made complaining such an art form that they

can brighten up a room by leaving it! Time and
time again I've seen people come into my practice
with their health in shambles. They feel absolutely
horrible all the time, and they tell me about it in
technicolor every time I am foolish enough to ask
them. No matter how much time I spend suggesting practical ways to *improve* their health and
the way they feel, they are more interested in
refining their litany of misery than in improving
the things they complain about. Sometimes the
best solution for people who don't want to get
better is for you to move on and invest your time
in people who are ready for change. Remember to
choose your friends wisely.

Your subconscious mind is crucial to your success in life, no matter what you set out to achieve
or become. You can take control over your subconscious mind by filling or "programming" yourself
with empowering thoughts. Each morning I recite
a key Bible verse to help myself begin on a positive
note: "This is the day the LORD has made. We will
rejoice and be glad in it" (Ps. 118:24). Then I try
to keep my mind and attitude focused on positive
things.

Pat yourself on the back every once in a while.
Tell yourself how well you are doing. (I'm not
talking about some kind of "pride" program. I
want you to develop a balanced, God-centered,
truthful self-image.) If you do this on a daily basis,

you will reprogram your mind toward the positive side of life. You will actually begin to feel better, look better, act better and do better.

Clinical studies have shown that cancer patients who have a proper mental attitude will do much better in their battle with cancer and all the mental baggage it brings. Do yourself a favor. Learn how to control your thoughts.

Keep Up Your Basic Maintenance

SOME OF THE body's most basic needs can be met free of charge with a great deal of personal satisfaction and benefit. Yet routinely we deprive our bodies of these essentials with the overworked excuse that we "don't have time" or that we "have things to do" (the same excuses we use to avoid regular exercise). These simple "maintenance" activities can quickly become vital when our bodies are injured or fall victim to a disease due to our negligence.

Until the Industrial Revolution upended the work habits of this country and other industrialized nations, little had to be said about the body's need for sleep. Most daily activities were ordered around the natural time divisions of day and night. People would simply rise with the sun—or just before sunrise if they lived on a farm where livestock-related chores had to be done early. Then the entire family would go to bed shortly after the sun went down. This was a practical necessity because artificial light could only be provided in limited measure by candles, oil lamps and torches. Open fireplaces handled most of the lighting and heating duties. Natural gas lamps and electric lights are relatively new phenomena in human history, first appearing in American homes in the late 1800s and early 1900s.

In our day, we often refer to the nearest large metropolitan area as "the city that never sleeps" or "where the lights never go out." Some people from larger cities make fun of smaller rural communities, saying, "They roll up their sidewalks at eight o'clock." (Many rural communities still set their social clocks to the natural rhythm of the sun, since agriculture is their primary industry.)

Most of us can name Fortune 500 companies whose manufacturing plants and administrative offices operate twenty-four hours a day, seven days a week, three hundred sixty-five days a year. The lights never go out, and the machinery never stops running unless a breakdown occurs. Many people in maintenance and service occupations adapt their lives to "shift work," with some unfortunate people working the "graveyard shift" (appropriately named). Such people hardly know what it is like to sleep when the sun is down. Their "day" may start around 10 P.M. and end at 6 A.M., just as the sun begins to rise. The effect that such a schedule has upon the human body can be devastating.

INVEST IN YOUR HEALTH

NOT ONLY IS it important to get an average of eight hours of sleep every twenty-four hours, but *how* you sleep is also important. If your mattress sags, then your spine is sagging, too! Find a way to buy buy a good mattress that is flat and firm. It is commendable to be a careful budgeter and money manager, but don't "save money" by living with something second- or third-best that directly affects your health every day! When it comes to a good mattress, don't hesitate to seek out and buy the best. You aren't investing in a mattress; you are investing in your health.

By the way, there is a right and wrong way to lie down at night when you sleep. Don't lie on your stomach when you sleep because it does terrible things to your back and respiration. Sleep on your side. Use three pillows. Put one pillow between your legs, put one underneath your arm and use the third pillow for your head. Avoid using overstuffed pillows that are too big for your head and neck. I use one of those new buckwheat-filled pillows for my head to provide maximum support. Make sure your head and neck remain at an angle that is close to their normal position to avoid getting a kinked neck. I strongly recommend that you avoid goose-down pillows, since they are one of the most prevalent sources of irritants for people who have dust allergies.

SLEEP WELL, LIVE WELL

IF YOU START an exercise program, you will quickly discover that you need a good mattress, and you will need to lie in the proper position at night. If you go to sleep with sore muscles on a poor mattress, you will wake up with sore muscles and even more stiffness and discomfort. Your body rebuilds damaged tissues and replenishes tissue fluids and nutrients while you sleep. You need to make sure your body gets enough rest to help this vital rejuvenation process. If you go to the trouble to learn how to sleep correctly, it will make a big difference in your health. If you don't sleep well at night, you won't be rested, and your body tissues won't recover well.

I learned these facts about proper sleep habits the hard way when I had to undergo back surgery to remove the L4/L5 disk from my back in 1988. The disk was damaged during the years I trained improperly with heavy weights while in my teens. When I was injured, I was confined to bed for months. That gave me a lot of time to figure out what worked and what didn't work while my back was healing. My spinal problems came along because I was trying to keep up with my friend Arnie in the gym. I didn't know any better. I was driven to meet certain goals as an athlete and weightlifter—and it almost cost me more than I could afford.

Goals are good, but goals that are given too high of a priority can be deadly. There are some things in life that are just more important than others. Put your time and effort where your heart is, and avoid the things that will rob you of your energy and your God-given purpose in life.

Please call my office for details on my Living in Divine Health tape series, which goes into more detail concerning this chapter.

PART II:
THE TOP TEN FOODS YOU SHOULD NEVER EAT

High-fat luncheon meat rank number one on the list of "Ten Foods You Should Never Eat."

Nine

AVOID THE CONCEALED DANGERS IN HIGH-FAT LUNCHEON MEAT

THERE ARE TEN foods you should never eat if you want to live a long, healthy and energy-filled life. This is my list of deadly foods, and it wasn't concocted on a whim; it is based on solid empirical research and decades of clinical medical histories detailing the treatment progress, lifestyles and diets of people fighting for their lives against cancer and other diseases.

Cancer is an immune system-related disease. In essence, we all "get cancer" every single day, but our own immune systems quickly search out and destroy these cancer cells under normal circumstances. We "get cancer" only when our immune systems break down or fail for some reason. (The activity of free radicals are the prime suspects in most cases.)

Once a diagnosis of cancer has been made, the

standard cancer-treatment protocols used in the
United States include surgery, chemotherapy, radiation treatments or a combination of the three.
Unfortunately, chemotherapy and exposure to
radiation therapy tend to weaken or compromise
the immune system, making it very difficult for
people to recover from cancer in some cases.[1]
When cancer patients ask me how to build their
immune systems, they are given "Ten Foods You
Should Never Eat" list.

High-fat luncheon meat rank number one on
the list. The list includes all pork products such as
bacon, sausage, ham, pepperoni and hot dogs.

RAISED ON WIENER SCHNITZEL, NEAR DEATH AT TWENTY-SEVEN

MAYBE YOUR RESPONSE is, "Oh, come on, Ted! We
love those foods. Our kids eat these foods all the
time. Most of them are lower in fat now, and they
really taste good!" I know what it is like to groan
over the need to give up pork products and
processed meats. My parents immigrated from
Germany in 1952. My first language was German,
and I was raised on sauerkraut, wiener schnitzel and
pork chops, plus mountains of hot dogs and
sausage and everything else ingenious Germans can
make with pork and pork by-products. (My dad
used to jokingly say to me, "Son, if you like

sausage, never watch us make it.")

Let me ask you a question: How did my childhood diet affect my health by the time I was twenty-seven years old? I told you that I nearly died of a heart condition, even though I was a highly conditioned athlete. How can I be sure my health problem had anything to do with pork products or high-fat luncheon meat? I know it did, because when I stopped eating pork and processed meats (and shellfish), my life-threatening heart problems quickly improved and ultimately disappeared—even though my doctors couldn't touch the condition with conventional antibiotics and other drug therapies.

It doesn't get any worse than pork. If there is one thing you learn from this book, let it be this: Don't eat pork. A pig is absolutely unfit for human consumption! It never has been fit, and it never will be. As far as I'm concerned, pigs were put here by God as scavenger feeders to help clean up the environment, but they were not put here for humans to eat.

Too Hot for the Body to Handle

ACCORDING TO CAREY Reams, a noted author and biochemist, one of the problems with pork and high-fat luncheon meat is that these foods digest too quickly in the human digestive system. They are literally too hot for the body to handle. They actually slow down the body's ability to fight off disease and cancer through the immune system. That makes it a big problem, because pork is used in a lot of foods most people overlook.

You might be surprised to learn that many people don't associate ham with pork. They just don't think about the connection. Most people don't realize that pork is the main ingredient in the number one pizza topping in America (and my former first choice as well)—pepperoni. You will recall that even as I was dying with a heart disease at age twenty-seven, I insisted on eating all the pepperoni slices my nutritionist friend, Jeff, had picked off of his pizza. I told him, "Jeff, I can't believe you're throwing away the best part!"

How ironic. I was dying of a heart disease that was probably instigated by my lifelong consumption of pork and high-fat luncheon meat like pepperoni, and I was telling Jeff he was throwing away the "best part." That sounds like Charlie Tuna telling the rest of the school of tuna, "Hey, the hook is the best part! I can't believe you're leaving it!"

I learned the hard way, but I don't want you to have to go through what I did. Avoid the high-fat meats and pork products. They are absolutely unhealthy. Let me give you several reasons why.

BACON—THE STRONGEST CARCINOGEN AROUND!

BACON, PERHAPS THE most popular pork product in the average grocery store, is loaded with sodium nitrite. This is the same preservative that appears in most high-fat luncheon meat. I am a biochemist, and thinking about what happens to sodium nitrite when it reacts with your stomach acids makes me very, very concerned. Do you know why? Sodium nitrite reacts with the powerful acids in your stomach to form *nitrosamines*—one of the most potent cancer-causing agents known to man.

It is no accident that the cancers affecting the digestive tract—particularly colon, pancreatic and stomach cancer—dominate the mortality charts. In my professional opinion, these deadly cancers are directly related to the high-fat foods we eat (many of which are "preserved" with sodium nitrite) and to the lack of fiber in the typical American diet.

As we learned in a previous chapter dealing with dietary fiber, meats literally can sit in the colon for extended periods of time (sometimes for weeks) before they are expelled from the body. This has clearly been associated with an increased risk of colon cancer. Smoked, pickled or salt-cured meats further compound the problem. Yet you will find them in abundance in the luncheon meat section of every grocery store in America.

The National Academy of Sciences issued a report warning the medical community and the American public that these processed meats contain two chemicals definitely shown to cause cancer in laboratory animals: nitrosamines (sodium nitrate) and polycyclic hydrocarbons. These chemicals are used in the processing of these meats and should be avoided, especially if you have a low-fiber diet. The association between these chemicals and cancer is so strong that it would be foolish to dismiss this warning given by the National Academy of Sciences in 1982.[2]

Again, I personally believe that pork is not fit for human consumption, even if the animals are fed grain and raised on sparkling clean floors. Pork, pork products and high-fat luncheon meat should be avoided at all costs.

HAVE YOU HAD YOUR
DAILY DOSE OF HOMOTOXIN?

WHY IS PORK getting such rough treatment by a prestigious research institute? In a clinical article titled "The Adverse Influence of Pork Consumption on Health," German Professor Hans-Heinrich Reckeweg, M.D., wrote:

Pork should be regarded as an important *homotoxin* (human poison), which initiates activation of the body's defense mechanisms. These defensive measures then manifest themselves in a variety of illnesses. Furthermore, from published reports, it became apparent that several constituents of pork behave as homotoxins or as stress factors, hence, for them, the term "sutoxins" appeared justified.[3]

Next time you take a big bite out of that BLT sandwich, sausage biscuit or tasty bacon strip, remember that you are flirting with danger. What I am about to tell you may cause you to change your opinion about certain kinds of food. Professor Lettre, a pathologist at Heidelberg University, one of the top research universities in the world, conducted a unique experiment using radioactive isotope tissue labeling. It involved labeling specific foods with radioactive atoms or substances so their movements through the human body could be accurately traced.

Professor Lettre conducted experiments with "living-cell therapy" to test the theory that the animal tissues humans consume will ultimately migrate to a similar location in the body of its human host. His study showed that radioactively labeled animal tissues from key organs and glands, upon being absorbed by the body, generally migrate to the equivalent position where they belonged biologically in the animal that had been eaten.

Lettre's study uncovered patients who had eaten a great deal of bacon from the pig's neck. These patients showed typical fatty folds on the back of their own necks. I know this sounds far-fetched, but this is a research finding from Heidelberg University.

EAT A PIG, LOOK LIKE A PIG

THE SAME PHENOMENON was true of patients who regularly consumed bacon, which is derived from a pig's stomach area. They began to develop thick bulges of fat on their own stomach areas. Furthermore, people who ate ham, especially women, showed irregular deformation in the buttock and hip areas, never realizing that ham was the cause. Basically the findings are saying, "If you want to look like a pig, eat a pig." I mean, come on, do you really want to go there?

The New Testament contains an interesting passage that describes a vision received by the apostle Peter approximately ten or fifteen years after Jesus' resurrection. The tenth chapter of the Book of Acts records the story of Peter's vision, when he saw a sheet being lowered from heaven that was filled with some of the animals the Bible classifies as "unclean" foods:

He saw the sky open, and something like a large sheet was let down by its four corners. In the sheet were all sorts of animals, reptiles, and birds. Then a voice said to him, "Get up, Peter; kill and eat them."

"Never, Lord," Peter declared. "I have never in all my life eaten anything forbidden by our Jewish laws."

The voice spoke again, "If God says something is acceptable, don't say it isn't." The same vision was repeated three times.

—Acts 10:11–16

What was Peter's response? "'Never, Lord,' Peter declared. 'I have never in all my life eaten anything forbidden by our Jewish laws'" (Acts 10:14). Peter was still following God's dietary principles years after Christ had been resurrected. What does that mean? If you turn to Acts 10:28, you will see where Peter says, "You know it is against the Jewish laws for me to come into a Gentile home like this. But God has shown me that I should never think of anyone as impure [or unclean]." In other words, Peter's vision had nothing to do with animals. The animals were used purely as symbols to illustrate a deeper truth concerning the equality of all mankind in God's eyes.

God did not send Christ to sanctify pigs—it didn't happen. We have convinced ourselves that it is OK to eat the only living animal Jesus ever killed according to Bible evidence. In Mark 5:13, He sent demons into a herd of swine, and two thousand pigs plunged to their death. Jesus didn't even bat an eyelash, even though the local pork farmers were so outraged because their source of commerce had been destroyed that they asked Jesus to leave the region. How could Jesus, who miraculously fed five thousand people and then warned his disciples not to waste any of the scraps, be so unfeeling about "wasting" two thousand pigs? The answer is simple: He did not consider the pigs to be a food source. He knew pigs shouldn't have been raised there anyway.

Actually, there was a big pit outside of Jerusalem where the townspeople threw all their garbage and excrement. Jerusalem didn't have running water or toilets in those days, and there were too many people for the city to follow the usual sanitary procedures of burying bodily excrement. The solution was to confine all human excrement in buckets, which were then dumped into the pit outside the city boundaries. Guess what was waiting at the bottom of Jerusalem's refuse pit looking for their next meal? Pigs.

The physical, biochemical and biblical problems with pork are bad enough, but we make matters worse with the chemicals we use to process the stuff. Remember, cancer is the leading cause of death among children who are fourteen years old or younger—except for accidents. You may be shocked to know that the United States has the highest infant-death rate of any industrialized nation on the face of the earth![4] The reason these statistics have become so grim is that in many cases we start off our lives with poor prenatal nutrition, followed by even worse childhood nutrition, which then manifests itself in the highest degenerative disease rates of any industrialized country. For our adults, *what is wrong with this picture?*

DOUBLE YOUR TROUBLE WITH NITROSAMINES

ONCE AGAIN, THE active carcinogen in hot dogs, luncheon meat and sausage is sodium nitrite. This chemical is so lethal that a pregnant woman can increase the risk of brain cancer in her infant by eating hot dogs. Why are these products still on our grocery market shelves? The sad truth is that we have some serious health problems in this country that are pretty much going unaddressed by the federal government. We need to realize that our health is our most valuable asset and that our health is our own responsibility. No one cares about your well-being and the well-being of your loved ones as you do, so the ultimate responsibility is yours. I heard an old Baptist preacher say one time that every pot sits on it own bottom.

Another reason to avoid high-fat luncheon meat may be the percentage of rat or rodent hair that can appear in the sausage and luncheon meat you eat. I do not want to do this, but I have to break the news to you that rats do not get hair cuts. They do not have access to barbers. The way you get your minimum daily requirement of rat hair is for an entire rat to fall into the grinding vats. So the next time you go to a ball game and order a corn dog, you may as well order a rat on a stick! (I hope you're not eating breakfast.)

You may have guessed by now that I am not your average nutritionist. Sometimes I feel like a cross-eyed discus thrower. I may not set any records, but I will definitely keep the crowd alert! My point with all of this is that rats are unhealthy; therefore, hot dogs are unhealthy.

"WHAT DID THE DOCTORS TELL YOU TO EAT?"

SEVERAL YEARS AGO, I met a young girl in the baggage claim area at Orlando International Airport who was returning to the Mayo Clinic. She was only eight or nine years old, and she was wearing a ski cap. I knew why she was wearing the cap when I saw that she didn't have any hair, so I asked her, "May I ask you what kind of problems you have?"

"Well, I have cancer," she said. "I've been at the Mayo Clinic undergoing cancer therapy."

"What have the physicians told you about what you should and shouldn't eat?" I asked.

She shrugged and said, "They told me to eat anything I want to eat. They said it doesn't matter what I eat, because food has nothing to do with cancer."

I looked at that precious little girl and said, "That's their opinion, but let me ask you a question: What foods do you eat?"

She looked up at me with her beautiful eyes and said, "All I eat are Twinkies, Ding Dongs, some hot dogs and diet sodas. That's it."

I thought to myself, *No wonder this girl has cancer. How in the world is she supposed to support her own immune system so that her body can recover from cancer when she is eating that kind of junk?* I am sad to say that counsel she received reflects the general nutritional ideas most common in this country.

Another one of my colleagues tells me this account: There was a ten-year-old boy who was diagnosed with bone cancer and had his left leg amputated. The boy's parents asked their doctor, "What caused this?"

The doctor shook his head and said, "Well, we don't know what caused it."

The parents then asked, "Do you think nutrition could play a role in this?"

The physician confidently told them, "Oh, no. Nutrition has nothing to do with your son's cancer."

Ask yourself this question, *If the doctor already said he didn't know what caused the boy's cancer, stating that he didn't have any idea about the cause of the cancer, then how could he so confidently rule out nutrition?*

WE HAVE A PROBLEM WITH FLAT-EARTH THINKING

ONLY FIVE HUNDRED years ago or so, the leading scientific minds of the age universally confirmed that the earth is flat. Anyone who disagreed with them faced excommunication and possible death. (Some of the early astronomers whom we revere today faced threats of excommunication if they held to their then-radical theories about the earth being "round.")

We all have "flat spots" in our thinking where it is easier to dismiss things that challenge our established viewpoints. The problem with the tendency of many healthcare professionals to dismiss poor nutrition as a factor in disease is that medical statistics and disease patterns say otherwise. We are leading the world when it comes to heart disease, diabetes and cancer, despite the fact that we also lead the world in medical technology and skilled medical care! Something is seriously wrong with this picture.

Virginia Livingston-Wheeler, M.D., established

the Livingston Foundation Medical Center in San Diego, California, in 1969. Her research and unconventional theories about disease prevention and cancer treatment through revitalization of the human immune system were dismissed and criticized by some members of the medical profession at that time.

The Foundation's cancer clinic and innovative Immunotheraphy cancer-treatment program have even been listed as a "quack treatment" for cancer by some groups (although without thorough documentation and with little or no reference to the program's success rates). These critics were embarrassed when respected mainstream researchers supported many of Dr. Livingston-Wheeler's theories and research findings through rigorous medical studies released in the orthodox journal, *Cancer*, published by the American Cancer Society.[5] Sometimes, you have to stick to your guns no matter what the "crowd" says:

Remember that pork products and high-fat luncheon meat are foods we definitely need to avoid. They are foods that aren't going to help us at all as far as maintaining a healthy body chemistry. They are foods that we would be a whole lot better off simply avoiding and not putting into our system whatsoever.

The risks greatly outweigh the culinary benefits of eating shellfish.

Ten

SIDESTEP THE HIDDEN HAZARDS OF SHELLFISH

SOME OF MY favorite foods (before my heart disease episode) occupy the "number two" position on the "Ten Foods You Should Never Eat" list. I am referring to shellfish, which includes lobster, crab, shrimp, oysters, scallops, mussels and clams, plus a subcategory of smooth-skinned amphibious and aquatic creatures that includes animals such as frogs, salamanders and eels.

There are three reasons I have eliminated these foods from my diet. First and foremost, I am inclined to exercise extreme caution any time God's Word warns mankind about particular foods. I am convinced there was, and is, more involved in the kosher food laws than mere religious separation. Second, the "Ten Foods You Should Never Eat" list is based on clinical research findings, not the personal diet opinions of one or two people. Third, this group of animals is being contaminated by environmental factors at an alarming rate, and they are passing along contaminants to everything and everyone that eat them.

Biologist and author Sandra Steingraber, Ph.D., is positive there is a direct link between eels who live in the cold waters of Canada's Lake Ontario near the contaminated lower St. Lawrence River and who migrate to the warmer Sargasso Sea in the Caribbean for mating and the beluga whales who live six hundred miles away in the uncontaminated St. Lawrence estuary. The beluga whales were suddenly struck by a mysterious cancer epidemic although they had no obvious exposure to contaminants. However, they *love to eat eels* that pass through their waters en route to their Caribbean spawning grounds.[1]

HOW ARE SHELLFISH CONTAMINATED?

IN SOME CASES, the probability of shellfish having toxemia or toxic problems may be low if they are farm raised or harvested in clean waters. Unfortunately, most of the fish species and algae on which shellfish feed migrate freely from one part of the ocean to the other, picking up poisons and chemical contaminants from the water and the things they eat along the way.

An especially important fact to remember is that

when something dies in an ocean or lake, its carcass will ultimately settle to the floor of that body of water unless a scavenger eats it first. It is common for sea life that passes through especially contaminated areas near industrial sites, chemical plants or large cities to become so toxic that they die. Sometimes it happens close to their contamination site, and sometimes it happens months later and thousands of nautical miles away. In any case, there are usually lobsters and other scavenger crustaceans waiting to clean up the mess by eating it.

This explains why the flesh of so many species of shellfish are found to be contaminated with mercury, lead, arsenic, carcinogens and hundreds of synthetic and chemical contaminants. You don't have to be a biochemist to realize that such contaminants can make these creatures toxic as well.

Shellfish need to be avoided. Some people have known this for centuries. My Jewish friends say, "Well, we told you so. Doesn't the Torah (in the Old Testament) expressly forbid the eating of pork and shellfish?" They are referring to the passages in Leviticus that specifically warn the Jewish people not to eat smooth-skinned fish, shellfish, pork or blood products:

> As for marine animals, you may eat whatever has both fins and scales, whether taken from fresh water or salt water. You may not,

however, eat marine animals that do not have both fins and scales. You are to detest them, and they will always be forbidden to you. You must never eat their meat or even touch their dead bodies. I repeat, any marine animal that does not have both fins and scales is strictly forbidden to you.

—LEVITICUS 11:9–12

When my Christian friends hear me talk about the dangers of eating pork or shellfish, they often ask me, "Are you trying to tell us that we are not going to get to heaven if we eat pork or shellfish?"

Invariably I tell them, "Absolutely not! You will get to go to heaven all right—*you will just get there a lot faster.*" I'm joking with them of course (well, sort of), but I still tell them to avoid pork and shellfish.

SOMETIMES PURE TROUBLE TASTES GOOD

LET ME CLARIFY the fact that we should avoid shellfish, but I did *not* say avoid seafood. Fish is an excellent choice for a low-fat, high-energy diet. Grouper, red snapper, orange roughy and salmon are all fine food sources—but avoid shellfish. You should also remember that I am not saying that lobster and shrimp don't taste good. These foods may taste good, but they are pure trouble when it comes to your physical health.

In 1981, when I had only been out of college for about one year, a friend of mine, Henry Minks, invited myself and my best friend, Gene Dawes, to dinner at an exclusive country club. It was an "all-you-can-eat" seafood buffet—with mounds of crab, lobster, shrimp, oysters, anything you could imagine. (I have since renamed such buffets as "make-a-complete-pig-out-of-yourself-and-eat-until-you're-miserable" buffets.)

My friends and I ate as if there were no tomorrow—and boy, did that food taste great. But we paid a miserable price for choosing poorly. I have never been as violently nauseated and ill—for five full days—in my entire life. My friends suffered the same fate. To this day I never knowingly touch shellfish.

Let's do a reality check. If God Himself said, "Don't eat it," don't you think He has already figured out our best diet? After all, we were created in His image.

In all fairness, some authorities make a distinction between the two classes of shellfish—those that move and those that do not. Dr. Dean Ornish, the author of *Eat More, Weigh Less,* strongly favors the purely vegetarian diet. His view of the matter differs from mine in several respects:

The ones [shellfish] that don't move, such as clams, mussels, scallops and oysters, are the vegetarians of the sea, and they consume the phytoplankton, or sea vegetables. Since these shellfish eat a vegetarian diet, their bodies are relatively low in fat and cholesterol. So, as Dr. William Castelli of the Framington Heart Study is fond of saying, "If you can't *be* a vegetarian, then *eat* a vegetarian."[2]

Other respected nutritionists would agree with Dr. Ornish in this area. However, the *focus* of their comments and recommendations tends to be upon the fat and cholesterol content of these foods. In that context, I would totally agree that shellfish, in general, are very low in fat and cholesterol and provide a high concentration of proteins and other necessary nutrients.

My focus, however, is upon the carcinogenic (cancer-causing) and pathogenic (disease-causing) components embedded in the flesh of these carnivorous scavengers and "filter-feeders" of the sea. An oyster can filter up to fifty gallons of sea water daily. No one needs these deadly ingredients in their diets.

Many of the shellfish varieties named above show up in major news releases year after year as being infected with deadly viruses, bacterial agents and chemical contaminants. These factors only heighten the biblical warnings God gave us about foods to be avoided.

PARALYTIC SHELLFISH POISON

As I WAS completing the final draft of this book, the Alaska Department of Environmental Conservation closed Kachemak Bay, a favorite harvesting site for commercial shellfisherman, after yet another outbreak of PSP, or paralytic shellfish poison. If it sounds deadly, that is because it is. State health officials there issued a report three years ago documenting one hundred seventeen outbreaks of sickness from PSP since 1973. One official said, "The toxin can be present at any time in Alaska marine environments." The Department's news release said:

> Paralytic shellfish poisoning comes from algae that are a food source for filter-feeding shellfish like clams and mussels. The shellfish store the toxin from the algae in their tissues. The toxin can be present even when there is no visible discoloration, or so-called 'red tides' in the ocean water. There is no home test outside the laboratory that is accurate in determining the presence of PSP. The toxin has also been found in crab viscera in recent years...
>
> Symptoms of PSP may appear soon after ingestion, perhaps in less than an hour. Initial symptoms commonly are a tingling or numbness in the lips and tongue, often

followed by tingling and numbness in the fingertips and toes. These symptoms may progress to loss of muscle coordination.

Other symptoms may be dizziness, weakness, drowsiness and incoherence. While there is no antidote for the toxin, it is important that vomiting be induced at the first sign of the onset of symptoms, and medical attention should be sought. Death can result from respiratory paralysis within twelve hours of eating PSP contaminated clams.[3]

Sometimes it isn't safe to "eat a vegetarian."

TOSS THE LOBSTERS, SPARE THE CATS

I'LL NEVER FORGET a time in the Florida Keys when I was preparing to go diving. When the previous client's boat came in with a fresh catch of lobsters, I watched the divemaster pull lobster after lobster out of large buckets, break off the lobster tails (which contain most of the edible meat) and throw the heads back into the water.

Behind this man were dozens of cats begging for the lobsters. It looked as if the dive ship supported the entire cat population of the Keys. This was so intriguing that I had to ask the man, "Why don't you feed these lobster heads to the cats instead of throwing them back in the water?"

"Oh, no," he said, "we can't give them to the cats. The poison in the lobsters will kill the cats." Hello?

Let me paint another picture to help burn this indelibly into your synapses. Picture two color photos in your mind. The first picture is of a large lobster—an arthropod. The second picture is of a very large cockroach, which is also an arthropod. What is your normal reaction to the arthropod we call a cockroach? Now picture the lobster in your mind and think, *A lobster is nothing more than a giant aquatic cockroach swarming on the bottom of the ocean.* There is at least a good chance that you will never look at a lobster in the same way. Again, God knows what He is doing, and in His Word He warned us about shellfish like the lobster.

You may still be protesting, "Oh, I love lobster, fresh snow crabs and soft-shell crabs when they are in season. I love that spicy Louisiana crayfish and giant Gulf shrimp from the bottom of the ocean. They taste so good." Several years ago after speaking for a crowd of fifteen thousand people in Miami, my wife and I were asked by my dear friend Peter Lowe, who had hosted the event, to have dinner with him and President Bush. There were only seven of us at this incredibly formal gathering. During the course of the conversation, we were able to ask President Bush anything we wanted. I asked him why Ross Perot disliked him so intently. After he had answered my question, he began asking me about nutrition and why snow crabs were so bad for you. After I answered his question, he simply smiled and the conversation turned to another topic. So I can honestly say that even if the president of the United States asks me a question about shellfish, I will tell him as I have told you. *Don't eat them.*

I'll be honest with you. I used to like them, too; in fact, the word *like* is probably too weak. I loved them, but a personal health crisis and two decades of research have led me to change my tastes forever. We need to remember that the shellfish "that move," such as crabs and lobsters, are flesh-eaters; they are not picky eaters. They will eat the decomposed flesh of diseased carcasses just as quickly as they will eat the flesh of living prey, and there is plenty of decomposed material on the bottom of the sea. This is how their bodies collect all the toxins, contaminants and waste products brought to them by the globe-circling currents of the sea.

LOBSTERS: THE "TYPHOID MARYS" OF THE SEA

DR. SANDRA STEINGRABER, herself a cancer survivor and researcher, said something that we all need to consider next time we think about ordering a plate full of mollusks or lobster:

Aquarium studies in the laboratory show that the same carcinogens known to cause cancer in humans and rodents also cause cancer in fish and mollusks—and they are often metabolized in the same way. Concordance is not perfect, however, and plenty of exceptions exist. Lobsters, for example, do not get cancer; they seem able to sequester carcinogens in their tissues in a way that prevents damage to their chromosomes.[4]

Don't rejoice over the fact that lobsters don't get cancer. Think of them as a type of aquatic "Typhoid Mary," a carrier of a deadly disease that devastates those with whom they come in contact, while leaving them untouched to carry their deadly cargo to its next unfortunate destination. To quote biochemist George Baily of Oregon State University, "Cancer is cancer is what we're finding out at the molecular level."[5]

FILTER-FEEDERS OR SEPTIC TANKS?

ANOTHER CLASS OF shellfish is filter-feeders; these are especially susceptible to water contaminants. These are the type that do not move, and they include clams, mussels, scallops and oysters. In a sense, they are one of the primary septic tanks in the ocean although they feed almost exclusively on water-borne plant matter. The problem is that to get the algae and plant matter (which can also be contaminated), they have to filter out everything else that floats by. They are not designed to be consumed by humans, period. That is not why God put them here.

The Smithsonian Institution and the National Cancer Institute jointly sponsor the Registry of Tumors in Lower Animals currently housed on the campus of George Washington University in Washington, D.C. The Registry holds thousands of specimens along with carefully preserved slides of the tumors removed from the specimen collection. You will find cancerous fish livers, clams with genital cancers and salamanders with skin cancer (another food we are not to eat). The Registry was founded to study the tumors that have begun to show up in cold-blooded fish, amphibians and reptiles, and those in other creatures such as corals, crabs, clams, snails and oysters.

The Registry has been very busy, and the accusing finger points directly toward environmental contaminants. Author and biologist Sandra Steingraber, Ph.D., wrote in her landmark book, *Living Downstream:*

> The preponderance of cold-blooded animals with cancer are aquatic bottom feeders. And the dark beds of rivers, lakes, and marine

estuaries are precisely where the highest concentrations of contaminants are found...

Adhering to fine particles of sediment and
pulled to the bottom by gravity, these chemicals slowly accumulate. Scavenger fish and
detritus-grazing mollusks are thus highly
exposed. They are also the animals most
severely afflicted by tumors.[6]

I live in Florida where fresh seafood is abundant
and very popular. Several times a year news
announcers on television will announce, "So-and-
so has died of toxic shellfish poisoning or paralytic
shellfish poisoning." Usually it happens when
people eat contaminated shellfish harvested from
contaminated waters during "red tide" (an annual
invasion of a particular kind of algae) or because
they ate it out of season. All I know is that it happens a lot.

"DON'T EVEN TOUCH THEM"

ONE OF THE most significant shellfish dangers to
arise in recent years, related primarily to oysters,
clams and mussels, is a bacterium named *Vibrio vulnificus*. This bacterium is in the same family as the
bacterium that causes cholera, but it thrives in warm
sea water (which is found along the entire Gulf
Coast and much of the Eastern seaboard facing the

Atlantic Ocean). This family of *vibrios* is called "halophilic" because they require salt to survive.

This bacterium can cause disease in people who eat contaminated seafood, and it is so virulent that it can infect people who expose an open wound to sea water or infected seafood. This is especially dangerous for fish industry workers and food pre-parers because cuts, nicks and abrasions are very common when attempting to open freshly har-vested clams without protective gloves. The Centers for Disease Control and Prevention (CDC) warns:

> *V. vulnificus* can cause disease in those who eat contaminated seafood or have an open wound that is exposed to sea water. Among healthy people, ingestion of *V. vulnificus* can cause vomiting, diarrhea and abdominal pain. In immunocompromised persons, par-ticularly those with chronic liver disease, *V. vulnificus* can infect the bloodstream, causing a severe and life-threatening illness character-ized by fever and chills, decreased blood pressure (septic shock) and blistering skin lesions. *V. vulnificus* bloodstream infections are fatal about 50 percent of the time.[7]

The CDC report also said that a recent study showed that people with preexisting medical conditions were eighty times more likely to develop V. vulnificus bloodstream infections than were healthy people. Doctors typically treat this condition with an antibiotic like Doxycycline or Ceftazidime.

One of the problems connected with this bacterium is that it does not alter the appearance, taste or color of oysters. Even oysters that are legally harvested in waters free of fecal contamination may be contaminated with *V. vulnificus.* Once again, the wisest course seems to be abstinence from these particular foods. The risks greatly outweigh the culinary benefits of eating shellfish.

YOU CAN'T EAT HIGH-
FAT, CHEMICALLY
PRESERVED JUNK FOOD
ON A REGULAR BASIS
AND BE HEALTHY.

Eleven

LEAVE YOUR
"JUNK" BEHIND

WHEN I WAS a little kid, I used to eat pork rinds and drink sodas all the time. I thought they were great. After all, they were crunchy, and they tasted good. Today I think it is sad because I didn't know any better. I would come home from school every afternoon, drag out my pork rinds (deep-fat-fried pork fat) and make myself several peanut butter and jelly sandwiches.

My mother was an immigrant from Germany who was used to all the high-fat foods and pork products for which Germany is famous, and she really didn't know anything about nutrition. It wasn't something that was taught in Germany—or in the United States—in those days. My mother never told me anything about what I should or should not eat, and it wasn't really an issue. She kind of let my sister Lois and I do the shopping, and you can image what we brought home.

My wife, Sharon, grew up in much the same way. Her father was a colonel in the Air Force, and Sharon was allowed to go to the base commissary and buy whatever she wanted. Naturally, she filled up on Little Debbies, Twinkies and cupcakes. When I met her, Sharon's blood sugar levels were so high that she probably should have already been put on insulin. It wasn't long before I said, "Honey, we really need to do something here."

By that time, Sharon was eating four to six candy bars a day.

I remember that the first night I went out with her, she ordered *two* hot fudge cakes. I learned that this was the way she ate every day. I watched Sharon devour all the chocolate-fudge covered ice cream and the fudge brownie underneath fairly calmly. Then she looked up at me with her beautiful eyes and said, "Do you mind if I get another one?"

I smiled and told her, "Have at it. You too will change."

By our third date, I proposed to Sharon. That was a pretty bold thing to do considering this young woman was eating all the things I had learned to avoid. I had just recovered from the problem with my heart, so I knew that if I was going to marry Sharon, then we were going to be eating right. She really wanted to be healthy, so she battled her way to freedom from her chronic junk-food addiction to become an expert on healthy cooking and food choices. In fact, she has put together one of the best health-food cookbooks on the market, and she is in the process of writing a book on children's nutrition.[1]

I'VE SEEN THE ETERNAL TWINKIE

SEVERAL YEARS AGO I saw a Twinkie at a health-food seminar sponsored by the National Health Federation in Orlando, Florida. That seemed kind of odd, but it was even more intriguing because this lone Twinkie package was sitting on a shelf by itself, looking as if someone had just purchased it at a local grocery store and had accidentally left it there that day. Finally I asked a man who stood nearby, "What is it with this Twinkie?"

"Well," he said, "we are trying to determine its shelf life. No one knows for sure just what that is."

My curiosity was getting the best of me, so I asked, "How long have you had it?"

I was shocked when he told me, "We have had it here at the seminar *for the past fifteen years.*" Think about the implications of that statement. The ingredients in that Twinkie are so void of nutrients that even God's common single-celled organisms and bacteria cannot get enough nutrients from it to sustain life—even over a fifteen-year span. Yet we feed the same stuff to our children in such amounts that a full 50 percent of their diet is composed of junk foods just like that lonely Twinkie (which, I presume, is still sitting on that shelf)! Then we wonder why America's children are having so many health problems.

You can't sustain life on junk food on a long-term basis. By junk food, I am referring to a very broad group of "foods" with some common characteristics. Nearly all junk foods are high in fat, sugar, salt and dangerous chemical preservatives. Prepackaged junk foods include all of the Little Debbie products, Twinkies, cupcakes, Moon Pies and hundreds of other confections just like them.

Another large category of junk foods includes almost every menu item offered by fast-food restaurants in the United States. I include all of the various fast-food burgers, sandwiches and potato products in my junk-food category for some very good reasons. These fast foods may lack some of the chemical preservatives found in prepackaged junk food, but they make up for it with the by-products of deep frying and charbroiling, which produces deadly hydrocarbon carcinogens that go directly into our bodies.

SAVOR THE SESAME SEEDS ON YOUR BUN

THESE QUICK-FRIED, deep-fried and charbroiled products are accompanied by a variety of high-fat sauces and highly acidic high-sugar additives and are sandwiched between doughy white bread buns containing extra doses of sugar. (One of the secrets of the "taste" you admire so much in these fast-food sandwiches is that they make sure a little extra sugar shows up in their hamburger and hot dog buns to please the picky palate.) Sesame seeds are sometimes added for an extra touch, which may well be the most nutritious part of the fast-food meal!

I also recommend that you avoid fast-food restaurants because you don't know what medium the restaurant uses to cook its fried food. Most fast-food restaurants use hydrogenated fats because they are plentiful, cheap and have what seems to be an eternal shelf life. This highly saturated fat is bad enough, but the problem is made worse by the fact that most of these restaurants rarely change the fats in their cooking oil vats because of the cost. The medical community has known for many years that once fat of any kind is heated to high temperatures for a period of time, *it undergoes a chemical transformation and becomes carcinogenic.* I don't know about you, but I'm not interested in eating an extra large "value pack" of carcinogenic deep-fried French fries with my carcinogenic diet cola.

You can't eat high-fat, chemically preserved junk food like pastries, pies, cakes, donuts, candy and sodas on a regular basis and be healthy. These foods have no nutrient density. In other words, you may get four or five hundred calories from a meal like that, but you probably won't get any vitamins, minerals or protein. You end up with a stomach full of calorie-laden food that has no nutrient value whatsoever.

There is a another class of junk foods that should probably be called "junk-food additives." One of the primary offenders in this category is MSG, or monosodium glutamate. You can purchase this highly addictive flavor enhancer right off the shelf in the spice areas of most grocery stories, despite the fact that it is very hard on the human digestive system. MSG, perhaps the spice of choice in Chinese cuisine and other Far Eastern foods, has been associated with allergy problems and many other health complications. Allergic reactions to MSG are most often characterized by breathing difficulties, chest pains, skipped heart beats and partial paralysis. Needless to say, most emergency medical technicians, emergency room physicians and certain Chinese restaurant managers are very familiar with the telltale signs of MSG allergic reactions.

HAVE YOU HAD YOUR GROWTH HORMONES TODAY?

ANOTHER PROBLEM IS that many of America's most popular fast-food chains may import their meats from sources outside the United States where *hormone additive levels* are not regulated by our standards. Many, if not most, animals raised for meat are given growth hormones to speed the rate of their growth between birth and the market. As a result, the level of hormones in the meat we consume can directly affect the levels of hormones in our bodies. This became very clear in Puerto Rico where two-year-old male and female children had developed female breasts equivalent to those of adult women due to the suspected hormone content of their food![2] Many of you may still remember the *20/20* exposé with Geraldo Rivera back in the 1980s concerning this topic.

Heart disease is the leading cause of death in the United States, claiming over a million victims per year. Thanks in a large part to our junk food fixation, more than 64 percent of all American males between the ages of forty and forty-nine are overweight! In contrast, only 31 percent of men in this age bracket in the Netherlands are overweight. The figure drops to 29 percent in Yugoslavia and 22 percent in Japan. (The men in that nation are starting to "catch up" with our rates of heart disease incidence because they are being Americanized by all of our fast foods and junk food.)

The medical community is concerned because atherosclerotic streaking—traditionally an indication of very advanced circulatory disease in older adults—is showing up in the bodies of three-year-old children! How can that be? These adult symptoms are already starting at that age because these children are living on high-fat, chemically laden foods like Twinkies, Ding Dongs, donuts, deep-fat-fried fast foods and hydrogenated oils.

ENROLL JUNIOR IN A JUNK FOOD DETOX PROGRAM!

IF THESE JUNK foods were only eaten once in a while as a treat, they probably wouldn't cause any harm to our children. But they aren't eaten once in a while; they often form the bulk of our children's diets. If we were to compare our children's junk-food intake with alcohol consumption, we wouldn't hesitate to enroll our kids in an emergency detoxification program!

Parents often defend themselves by saying, "That is all they want to eat." My question is this: Does a two-year-old really know what is good to eat and what is not good to eat? Is a two-year-old really going to like eating his vegetables? *No.* Should you give your two-year-old a choice? *No.* Sadly, a lot of people do.

A distraught mother called me from Texas to tell me between sobs, "My little boy is going in for surgery. He is only twenty-four months old, and he has been on an IV-feed for the last three months in the hospital. In two days, the doctors are going to remove his colon. The human resources people have gotten involved, and they are not even giving me a choice. Do you know of another gastroendocrinologist who could give me a second opinion and hopefully stop this from happening? We will have to get a court order."

You can see how serious this situation had become.

I said, "Well, Ma'am, offhand I don't know of a specialist like that in Texas, but I can give you the name of a health professional in California who could perhaps help you" (which I did). Then I said, "Before you get off the phone, I promise I will never use your name... but you have to answer one question for me: What were you feeding your child before this happened?"

This brokenhearted mother just broke down into tears. By this time she was sobbing uncontrollably, but she managed to say, "He only eats one of three different types of foods. He is still drinking breast milk [which was fine], but there are only two other types of food that he will eat—potato chips and candy."

I never heard from this lady again. I only hope and pray that she was able to correct the problem without surgery. Why is it in so many cases that we wait until some devastating disease ravages our family before we seriously consider healthy alternatives?

Avoid the Wonders of White Bread and White Flour

OUT OF NECESSITY, I have made my definition of *junk food* very, very broad. Even some of the "staple foods" that form the foundation of the traditional American diet fall under the term *junk food.* Perhaps you remember the television ads aired several years ago trumpeting the virtues of Wonder Bread. The ad slogan said, "Wonder Bread helps build bodies in twelve different ways!" I believe this was a reference to the twelve vitamins the manufacturer added to its "enriched bread" (they had to add nutrients since the majority of the natural nutrients had been bleached, leached and processed out of the "enriched" flour long before it reached the bakery).

White Bread Dodge Ball

WE USED TO take slices of Wonder Bread (although any commercially made white bread would do), peel away the crust and wad it up into dough balls. Then we used our fresh dough balls to play pitch or to bounce them off walls, ceilings and each other. The bread was so doughy that we could make some really hard balls that lasted quite a while and really made an impression on an opponent who wasn't paying attention. I didn't know it then, but that is exactly what white bread does inside the digestive system, too. What a wonder.

White bread is made with highly processed, bleached white flour (no bran or fiber left)—like most of the junk food that contains any bread in it. White flour is so devoid of nutrients that manufacturers have to add something to it to talk us into buying it. To get white, bleached, "enriched" wheat flour, you have to strip totally the wheat kernel of all its nutrients and fiber. Only the starchy middle section of the wheat kernel is used. Then you bleach out the flour so it is nice and white, add some inexpensive chemically synthesized vitamins (mostly petroleum-based and indigestible by the human body) and you can legally label it as "enriched flour" and make "enriched bread" with it.

We need to eliminate white bread and bleached, white "enriched" flour from our diets and replace it with unbleached whole-grain flour and breads. (I recommend Ezekiel Bread, based on the Old Testament recipe.) I am amazed every time I go to the grocery store, where I see line after line of grocery carts piled high with "enriched" white bread, "enriched" and thoroughly bleached white flour, white sugar, "enriched" white rice, and package after package of junk foods made with lard, partially hydrogenated oils, lots of sugar and chemicals and that "enriched" bleached white flour.

"THE GOVERNMENT WOULDN'T LET ME BUY SOMETHING UNHEALTHY"

IT SADDENS ME because most of those people sincerely believe they are eating well. I used to ask them questions about the food in their carts while I was waiting in those checkout lines, but I stopped doing that. When I did ask them why they still purchased white bread and junk-food products, they looked at me with an expression that said, "What are you talking about? Why shouldn't I eat white bread? I mean, the government wouldn't let me buy a product that wasn't healthy for me. It wouldn't say 'enriched' if it wasn't good for me."

The truth is that government regulatory agencies like the Food and Drug Administration are small agencies with a big job. They operate with limited budgets, limited manpower and limited authority to enforce their own rules. On top of that, they are staffed by very human people. There are a lot of so-called food products that the FDA has approved that are so unsafe they should never be allowed out of the laboratory that spawned them (many of these products are described in this book). Other very excellent products that should have been approved were not.

LET THE BUYER BEWARE

THE BILLION-DOLLAR industries that prepare and market most of the foods on our grocery shelves are in business for only one reason: to make money. Frankly, their stockholders pressure them to get as much money from the American public as they possibly can. Do you really think their corporate concerns about your health can compete with the costs of running manufacturing plants and technology upgrades? In most cases, the answer is no.

Some food manufacturers will market anything that will make money and squeak past the few regulatory agents who poke their heads inside their plants during a five-year period. That takes us back to the ancient warning, *Caveat emptor* ("Let the buyer beware").

We launched the second chapter of this book with a statement made by Dr. Richard Brannon, chairman of the Board of Trustees of the International Academy of Preventive Medicine: "Most of the food in America today will support life, but it won't sustain health." That statement accurately describes most of the food in America today. You can sustain life, but how about your health?

What if I said, "OK, here is what we are going to do. We are going to live on Twinkies, colas and cupcakes for the next six months"?

Would you be alive in six months? Yes. How do you think you would feel? I know a lot depends on your genetics, your reserve energy and other factors, but the chances are very good that you would not be very healthy or feel very good or have much energy. In fact, you might have begun to show the symptoms of some degenerative diseases stemming from the lack of nutrients in your diet.

America's kids are getting sicker primarily because 50 percent of the foods in their diet have no nutrient value. That means they have to make up 100 percent of their nutritional needs with the remaining 50 percent of the calories they consume.

The same thing happens to people on a thousand-calorie daily diet who suddenly decide to eat a fat-free pastry. Those things are delicious, but it backfires when people get in the habit of binging on those things. What you will do is end up eating a bunch of that stuff on a regular basis saying, "Well, it's fat-free, and my doctor said I could have it because it is fat-free." They end up getting too few nutrients from their food, and they try to make it up using supplementation with vitamins and minerals. This is not healthy.

What is healthy? If you need a fast snack, eat some fresh fruit on the run. Stay with more complex carbohydrates like lentils, beans, rice and whole grains.

AVOID HEALTH-FOOD JUNK FOOD

I HAVE PROBABLY unintentionally offended almost everyone I can think of except vegetarians, so my warning to you if you are a vegetarian is this: Stay away from the "health-food junk food" called *tofu*. A full 60 percent of the calories in tofu come from fat. It should have never been touted as a miracle food for vegetarians. It richly deserves its official designation in this book as junk food.

During one of the rare times when I turned on my television set, I watched as a television minister read a letter from one of his program's viewers. This viewer had written to say she was dying of cancer. She said all her friends had stopped visiting her because she was wasting away in a hospital bed. She had lost 40 percent of her body weight, and she looked so bad that even her best friends couldn't bear to come into her room. She was in such bad shape that her friends would just cry when they saw her. The only person she felt was still her friend was this television minister, and she would watch him regularly on TV. She explained that she didn't have a job, so she couldn't buy the calendar that he was giving away to viewers who were able to help support the program with monetary gifts. At the end of the letter she added that the primary reason she didn't have a job was because *she was only twelve years old.*

DON'T FEED YOUR KIDS JUNK

I DON'T THINK we realize what we are doing to ourselves and our children sometimes. Many times I tell the people who attend my health seminars:

> If you want to clog your arteries with choles-terol and fat because of your dietary choices, then have at it. It is your decision. We live in America, don't we? If you want to kill your-self on the installment plan by eating this kind of junk food, then go ahead and do it. I won't force you to eat right, and neither will God.
>
> No one is going to go home with you tonight and make you eat right. It is a deci-sion you have to live with. But I ask this favor of you from the bottom of my heart as a father... *please don't feed your kids the junk.* Don't put it in the house. Your three-year-old or your six-year-old is not going to go to the grocery store in his car, whip out his wallet and buy junk food. You are. You are the one bringing this poison home and feeding it to your children.

This may sound pretty hard, but most of the parents in these seminars know in their hearts that I am right (and all of them know my motive for saying these things). I don't have to press the point; most of them came to the seminars looking for answers because they want to live an abundant life marked by good health and long life. Junk food makes for bad health and an uncertain future. We can do better with just a little knowledge, effort and determination. I'm supplying a lot of the information. You must supply the effort and the determination.

MORE FOOD ALLERGIES
IN HUMANS HAVE BEEN
TRACED TO DAIRY
PRODUCTS THAN TO
ANY OTHER SOURCE.

Twelve

WEAN YOURSELF
FROM HIGH-FAT
DAIRY PRODUCTS

HIGH-FAT DAIRY products have earned the "number four position" in the "Ten Foods You Should Never Eat" list because they can actually increase your risk of acquiring certain types of diseases. Another reason is that 60 percent of the allergies afflicting people in this country are directly attributable to the consumption of dairy products. Still, that is not the worst of it.

Whole milk is second only to beef as the largest source of saturated fat in the American diet.[1] If you remember how dangerous a high-fat diet is to the human body, consider the fact that of all the calories provided by whole milk, 50 percent are in the form of highly saturated milk fat. Of the calories found in our favorite whole-fat cheeses, an unbelievable 70 to 90 percent of the calories come from the milk fat they contain. These are unhealthy products in anybody's vocabulary.

Tell me the truth: Did you feel a strong negative reaction when you read that dairy products were listed on the dreaded "Ten Foods You Should Never Eat" list? Why? It is because it goes against everything you were taught as a child! The answer to why we eat and drink so many dairy products today can be traced back to the 1950s and 1960s when the Dairy Council (along with such food-industry giants as Kellogg's, Del Monte and Pillsbury) first launched their joint public-relations campaign.

Their goal was to convince the population of the United States into believing that there were "four main food groups." Naturally we learned that we had to include the "milk group" among the essential food groups of life. That is simply not true, but when has that mattered in the wacky world of commerce and government?

Large colorful posters flooded virtually every elementary school in America. Magazine ads for the "Four Food Groups" showed up in everything from *Time* magazine to the *Journal of the American Medical Association,* and television ads filled the airways.

The revenues of the dairy industry went sky high as conscientious parents, dieticians, school cafeteria workers and healthcare providers made sure their beloved children all had their daily allowance of milk and dairy products. (Our allergies zoomed out of control as well! I've never researched it, but I suspect we could trace a sudden growth spurt in the medical specialty of allergist to that same time period.) The revenues stayed at high levels until the truth began to leak about about dairy foods and the dangers of a high-fat diet.

THE DREADED "DIETARY CALCIUM DEFICIENCY" IS A MYTH

THIS WELL-PLANNED media blitz succeeded in convincing parents and busy healthcare providers that milk was "nature's most perfect food." Dr. John McDougall, in an excerpt from his book *The McDougall Plan,* eloquently finishes the story:

> The possibility of developing some vague illness imagined as "dietary calcium deficiency" haunts those not consuming milk and milk products. However, calcium deficiency of dietary origin is a myth and is virtually unknown in humans, even though most people in the world do not consume milk after weaning. The whole truth is that dairy foods are the most harmful of the traditional four food groups. They are high in fat, protein and environmental contaminants and deficient in fiber and carbohydrates.[2]

God's Internal Markers

As a scientific researcher, I am firmly convinced that God created living things with instincts and with actual internal "markers" or physical indicators that help direct the food choices and life patterns of each species—including His highest creation, man. Dr. McDougall cites three different sources in medical literature that pinpoint what I feel is an unmistakable physical indicator, lactose intolerance:

> After the age of four years, most people naturally lose the ability to digest the carbohydrate known as lactose found in milk, because they no longer synthesize the digestive enzyme, lactase, which lines the small intestine. This condition, known as lactose intolerance, results in symptoms of diarrhea, gas and stomach cramps when lactose-containing dairy products are eaten. Lactose intolerance is especially common among adult blacks and Asians, occurring in as many as 90 percent of these people.[3]

Do I Have to Give Up the Cheese?

Whether you are lactose-intolerant or not, you may have made the decision to eliminate excess

saturated fats from your diet (and I strongly recommend it for maximum health and renewed
energy levels). I have to admit that it means you
will also need to eliminate most dairy products as
well. "But Ted, I really like cheese." I like cheese
too, but I can't eat it because it makes me gain
weight. Its high levels of saturated fat are very hard
on my heart and cardiovascular system. I had to
learn this the hard way, so I have greatly reduced
these foods from my diet.

Cow's milk really isn't necessary for human
health. As we've already shown, you will increase
your risks of heart disease if you drink whole milk
because of its extremely high-fat content. If you
really feel you have to continue drinking milk, I
recommend that you switch to *certified* raw goat's
milk. Avoid pasteurized goat's milk because many
of the enzymes have been destroyed by the high
heat of the pasteurization process. The purpose of
the certification is to ensure that you aren't getting
any contaminants in the goat's milk, and yet this
process doesn't reduce the milk to "bleached
water."

Certified goat's milk is so rich that you can
dilute it fifty-fifty with water, and it will still taste
very good. (We have found that canned goat's milk
acquires a disagreeable taste, so we don't recommend it to our clients.) Goat's milk is very close in
consistency and nutrient content to human milk,

and it is reasonably good for your body. My advice is that you eliminate most dairy products and cheeses with the exception of an occasional glass of raw certified goat's milk as a condiment or in cereal. (That is, only if you don't have a weight problem. If you do, you should eliminate milk of any kind altogether. If you are going to drink milk regardless, use skim milk if possible to help avoid the hormones and antibiotics added to regular milk.)

One exception to this rule against drinking whole milk would be for children under the age of two. Toddlers must take in enough dietary fat to ensure proper brain, nerve and myelin formation. Those are very important parts of the human body that are still being formed during the first two years of life. However, I again recommend raw certified goat's milk as a better alternative to cow's milk because it is a much better product for children, and it doesn't cause nearly as many allergy problems. It is considered much healthier for children because of the close similarities between goat's milk and human milk. In fact, goat's milk is often referred to as the "orphan's milk," since almost all mammals can be raised healthily on it.

In my opinion, if at all possible, infants should not be given formula—despite what the baby formula manufacturers say. The very best formula for babies is mother's milk, and this should be their source of nourishment for at least nine to twenty-four months. (In those instances when breastfeeding is impossible, I recommend using goat's milk. Again, I recommend coordinating your decisions in this area with your primary healthcare provider.) Baby formula is considered by many international health professionals to be a deadly curse for children in underdeveloped nations. One official maintains that bottle feeding of infants in underdeveloped countries, such as India, is "a virtual death sentence."[4]

Robert S. Mendelsohn, M.D., a noted pediatrician with thirty years of clinical experience, writes in his book, *How to Raise a Healthy Child...in Spite of Your Doctor:*

> Cow's milk is deficient in iron and should not be given to babies for at least six months. Even then it should be introduced with caution, because many babies—perhaps as many as 15 percent—are allergic to cow's milk. It should be suspected as the potential cause of many illnesses.[5]

Twenty-five Ways to Say, "I'm Bad for You"

MORE FOOD ALLERGIES in humans have been traced to dairy products than to any other source. More than twenty-five different proteins have been identified in dairy products that can make your body revolt in an allergic reaction.[6] Most of these allergic reactions are respiratory in nature, producing elevated levels of mucous, nasal stuffiness, runny nose, sinusitus, asthma-like symptoms and inner ear inflammations.

Some people experience skin irritations such as hives, rashes or more serious conditions. For instance, dairy products have been linked to at least 50 percent of childhood iron-deficiency anemia and an unknown percentage of anemia found in adults. Some studies indicate that dairy products can be contaminated with viruses that cause leukemia, as well as with lesser disease-causing bacterial agents such as *E. coli, salmonella* and *staphylococci*.[7] They have also been linked to the incidence of Hodgkin's disease.[8]

TEN YEARS...AND IT SEEMS LIKE YESTERDAY

ANOTHER SERIOUS PROBLEM with milk is that it is produced by cows that feed on hay grown in fields contaminated by banned pesticides more than a decade earlier! Biologist Dr. Sandra Steingraber describes this scenario in chilling detail:

Aldrin and dieldrin [pesticides] were banned in 1975, although aldrin was allowed as a termite poison until 1987. Aldrin converts to dieldrin in soil and inside our tissues. Dieldrin suppresses the immune system and produces abnormal brain waves in mammals. As late as 1986, dieldrin was still turning up in milk supplies because the soils of hayfields sprayed more than a decade earlier remained contaminated. Most agricultural uses of chlordane in the United States were ended in 1980 and heptachlor in 1983. Both have been linked to leukemia and certain child-hood cancers.[9]

On a more upbeat note, Dr. McDougall says that many Western Europeans who were suffering with diagnosed coronary artery disease (heart disease) in the 1940s made an eye-opening discovery as a result of the hardship of war:

During World War II many people in Western Europe with established heart disease (coronary artery disease) had to switch from a rich diet *high in dairy* and meats to a diet of grains and vegetables. The death rate in these countries from heart disease dropped dramatically during this forced dietary change. Many studies have demonstrated that a decrease in death rate from heart disease can result from a change to a low-fat, low-cholesterol diet.[10]

Most people experience a range of allergic symptoms to milk that are less painful than those of lactose-intolerance and less deadly than those described by Dr. Steingraber, but the symptoms are still uncomfortable. Nearly everyone who is allergic to dairy products will manifest their reaction in their behavior as well as in purely physical symptoms. They will tend to be irritable, restless, unusually hyperactive or lethargic, and they may complain of muscle pain or sink into mental depression.

"GIVE ME A GLASS OF MUCUS, PLEASE"

ON A LESS serious note, whenever I drink milk or eat dairy products, an unbelievable amount of excess mucus builds up in my system. This isn't the most serious symptom of a dairy allergy, but it may well be the most universal misery suffered by human consumers of dairy products.

The day after I eat ice cream, you might see me running around with a box of tissues under one arm as I blow my nose for twenty to thirty minutes in an effort to clear out all the mucus generated in the previous twelve hours! I know this is a "physical indicator" that I am allergic to milk products, because when I don't drink milk, I don't have this problem. Needless to say, milk is a powerful "mucus former" and should be avoided by most adults.

"I'LL TAKE AN AMYL ACETATE (BANANA FLAVORING) SPLIT, PLEASE"

ICE CREAM HAS been the downfall of many well-meaning and sincere commitments to healthier diets. If you are like me, then you can understand why. It is time for another confession: I still have a soft spot for good ice cream, so I give in to it once in a long while because I know that an occasional celebration (one to two per year) with rich foods won't hurt me.

If you are going to eat ice cream (and I know you probably will no matter what horror story I tell you), make sure you get the highest-quality ice cream you can find (this is true for any dairy product you feel you must eat). I recommend Breyers or Häagen-Dazs ice cream. A lot of the cheaper ice creams on the market contain extremely dangerous chemical substitutes for the real thing. This includes the synthetic chemical flavorings many manufacturers use, the kind of ingredients that you have trouble pronouncing, such as:

- *Benzyl acetate* is an artificial strawberry flavoring that is also a nitrate solvent.

- *Amyl acetate* is used as an artificial banana flavoring—as well as a powerful paint solvent!

- *Butyrlaldehyde* is used as an artificial nut flavoring. You will also find it in your rubber cement.

- *Ethyl acetate* is a popular artificial pineapple flavoring, and it also does double duty as a leather cleaner. Its vapors are known to cause chronic lung, liver and heart damage. (I suppose the theory is that it "won't hurt you" when whipped into ice cream.)

- *Pepernial* is used in place of vanilla for flavoring. This chemical is used to kill lice. (I didn't realize vanilla extract was that expensive. They sure haven't dropped the price of lice shampoos lately.)

- *Acetiel C17* is an aniline dye that is used in plastic, and it is popular with manufacturers because it gives ice cream a nice cherry flavor.

- *Diethylglycol* is a cheap chemical used as an emulsifier instead of eggs.

Just think about that. You get all of those high-tech chemicals thrown in every time you eat lower-priced processed ice cream from the store! If you have to give in to your cravings for ice cream, do it very rarely and make sure you get Breyers,

Häagen-Dazs or some other premium brand with an ingredients list that you can read and completely understand. Look for whole milk, cream, eggs, natural vanilla flavoring and sugar, but make sure there are no stabilizers, gums, artificial flavors or any fancy words that you can't understand. Basically, if you can't pronounce it, you probably don't need it. It wasn't created in nature; it was dreamed up in a test tube somewhere, and that is where it should remain.

AVOID ANYTHING WITH HYDROGENATED OR PARTIALLY HYDROGENATED VEGETABLE OILS.

Thirteen

THE HEART-STOPPING TRUTH ABOUT MARGARINE PRODUCTS

YOU ALREADY KNOW that I grew up on a "classic American diet" that consisted of peanut butter and jelly on white bread washed down with large glasses of whole milk. By the time I was in sixth grade at the age of eleven or twelve, I was overweight and suffering from the weighty social consequences.

Worst of all, I didn't understand why. No one ever told me that 60 percent of the calories in the best-selling brands of peanut butter come from fat and something called *partially hydrogenated fat* or *trans fats*. As a childhood survivor, let me tell you: If your children have a weight problem, give them a new lease on life by cutting out the peanut butter and other margarine and bread products.

Margarine and all margarine-like products managed to rank number five on my "Ten Foods You

229

Should Never Eat" list. I'm sure it wasn't easy, since there are so many unhealthy contenders out there, but this "trans-fat" family has really earned its bad reputation. How? Basically, the harder the margarine or shortening, the more highly hydrogenated it is. The main problem with the hydrogenation process is that it causes trans fats to act somewhat like saturated fats in terms of their effect on blood cholesterol levels, but with some very dangerous side effects.

The *New England Journal of Medicine* published a study on the relationship between women's fat intake and the risk of heart disease. The study, conducted by researchers from Harvard School of Public Health and Brigham and Women's Hospital over a fourteen-year period studied more than eighty thousand individuals who had no history of coronary disease, stroke, cancer, high cholesterol or diabetes.

The study found that "a higher dietary intake of saturated fat and trans-unsaturated fat was associated with an increased risk of coronary disease, whereas a higher intake of monounsaturated and polyunsaturated fats was associated with a decreased risk."[1] The researchers concluded that replacing saturated and trans fats with unhydrogenated monounsaturated and polyunsaturated fats is more effective in preventing heart disease in women than reducing overall fat intake.

Another study indicated that trans fats may raise LDL cholesterol to *even higher levels* and *increase the risk of coronary heart disease.*[2] At least one study has linked breast cancer risk with high levels of trans-fatty acids in adipose tissue.[3] One thing is clear: Saturated fatty acids (except stearic acid) raise total and LDL-cholesterol levels and increase your health risks.

WHERE DID MARGARINE COME FROM?

MARGARINE WAS DEVELOPED in the United States during World War II when there was a shortage of butter. Food processors discovered that they could heat an oil such as vegetable oil, which was readily available and inexpensive, and pump liquid hydrogen through it to form a "hydrogenated" oil that was solid at room temperature. Biochemists call these *trans fats* because they are in transition. (Some trans fats occur naturally in certain meats and dairy products.)

This new product met a temporary need during the war, but manufacturers liked the product because trans-fatty acids like margarine and Crisco have a longer shelf life—a *much longer shelf life*— than unhydrogenated oils. They felt that the hydrogenation process created a more stable liquid or semi-solid form, which better suited their marketing goals. They noticed that hydrogenated vegetable oils like margarine are more spreadable than traditional refrigerated butter, so it could be used immediately upon removal from the refrigerator. Some manufacturers also claimed their partially hydrogenated vegetable oil shortenings made flakier pie crusts than butter or oils. The partial hydrogenation process increased the stability of oil in the sense that it made it less susceptible to spoiling when exposed to air. The rest is marketing history.

The problem with partially hydrogenated vegetable oils is a familiar one—we have taken natural foods and altered them into man-made substances that the body cannot handle. These *trans fats* can block what are called "LDL receptors" (LDL cholesterol is the "bad" cholesterol—these receptors actually receive or intercept dangerous cholesterol particles). The result may be significantly raised LDL and cholesterol levels in the body, which can be precursors of cardiovascular disease, heart attacks, strokes and a host of other serious health problems. This could explain why margarine consumers have a *higher incidence of heart disease* and *cancer* than the general population!

The hydrogenation process involves forcing hydrogen atoms into the holes of healthy unsaturated fatty acids to make them solid at room temperature (and in your blood vessels as well). This is done with hydrogen gas under pressure with a metal catalyst (usually nickel) at a temperature of 248–410 degrees Fahrenheit. Manufacturers do this because vegetable oils are liquid and too soft to be sold in stick or tub form. Saturated fats like pure butter and stearic acid (found in red meats) are too hard. Margarine requires something in the middle, so manufacturers add only enough hydrogen atoms to reach the perfect marketable consistency. Unfortunately, this does dangerous things in the manufacturing process while producing what we know as margarine and partially hydrogenated vegetable oil products like Crisco and shortening.

THE WORST PART OF IT ALL

THE INCOMPLETE HYDROGENATION process used by margarine manufacturers leaves unsaturated fatty acids in transition, with some of its molecules hydrogenated and some that are not. Author and researcher Udo Erasmus writes, "So many different compounds can be made during partial hydrogenation that they stagger the imagination. Scientists have barely scratched the surface of studying changes induced in fats and oils by partial hydrogenation."[4]

The worst part of it is that many of the altered substances produced by the partial hydrogenation process are toxic to our systems. One study has shown that up to 60 percent of the content of some margarines are trans-fatty acids, with less than 5 percent of the original essential fatty acids surviving the manufacturing process. The *average trans fat content* of stick margarines is 31 percent.

Despite all these facts, margarine is still praised as the savior of uninformed health-minded, fat-conscious people by its manufacturers (who know better) and by health practitioners who often have little nutritional training and even less time to pursue the truth through their own research. The reason most people believe margarine is a "heart-healthy" substitute for butter is because of the gross misinformation and deception in the marketplace.

Although many people in the health and nutrition fields, including myself, have been telling people about the dangers of margarine and margarine products for nearly twenty years, even more people have been saying otherwise until now. Time and time again, spokespersons have made bold statements about the dangers of butter while citing "independent studies" (independent in the sense that they were usually commissioned and conducted by margarine manufacturers) "proving" that margarine is the best way to go.

We no sooner counteract one bit of misinformation with solid scientific fact than news outlets around the nation announce other studies by organizations like the American Heart Association warning the American public to cut cholesterol at any cost. Their warnings come with an urgent plea to "cut out the butter and use margarine." Inevitably, other studies conducted at a slower pace by equally respected medical institutions will come to light, which say, "No, that is all wrong. Butter is better; margarine is bad" (although these reports generally get much less press).

WHO SAID THAT?
(AND WHAT IS THEIR MOTIVE?)

THE ONE THING we should always remember is this: *Consider carefully the source* of any research study you read or hear about in the health or food arena. In particular, make sure that studies trumpeting the virtues of manufactured foods have not been paid for by the companies marketing those products. I've found that even our most prestigious medical societies, health associations and leading government officials will sometimes lend their considerable weight to the erroneous claims of manufacturers or marketers (hopefully because their staff members are too busy to do their own independent research). The history of the U.S. Food and Drug Administration (FDA), for instance, is allegedly filled with unfortunate stories of alliances with the very industries that department was created to regulate.[5] Fortunately, the truth about trans fats, margarine and partially hydrogenated vegetable oils is finally beginning to leak out to consumers.

If you look closely at the margarine shelf in your local grocery store, you will probably find one or two major brands of margarine featuring a bold banner that says, "NO TRANS FATS." I still don't recommend those products because of the other junk put in them, but this is just the beginning. There is a new awareness in the medical and research community that *trans fats*—margarines or partially hydrogenated vegetable oils—are very dangerous for your health.

IF WE GET WHAT WE WANT, WE LOSE

WHAT MANY PEOPLE *do not know* is that margarine products containing high levels of trans fats include such popular products as Jif and Skippy peanut butter, prepackaged cake icings, candy bars of all types and descriptions and virtually anything that requires what is termed as a "smooth mouth feel." This term describes the sensation and texture that fat produces on the tongue.

Manufacturers have known for a long time that this creamy, smooth and slightly "thick" feel on the tongue actually determines how much people like certain foods. This explains why there are so many "thickeners, texturizers and fillers" on our food labels and in our food. We rate one ice cream or cake mix better than another because of the "creamy feel" we sense as it melts on our tongue. In the case of trans fats, if we get what we think we want—we lose.

How Old Is Your Wedding Cake?

THE THEME OF this chapter is really pretty simple: Avoid anything with hydrogenated or partially hydrogenated vegetable oil. Just to show why I am so determined to wean you from margarine products, let me tell you about my visit to a wedding shop in Tallahassee, Florida, a few years ago. I noticed several wedding cakes that were on display in a nonrefrigerated big glass case. I went to the lady in charge and said, "These wedding cakes are beautiful. Are they real, or are they just store displays?" The lady shook her head and assured me, "Oh no, these are actual wedding cakes. They are definitely real."

"That is interesting," I said. "What is the icing made of?"

She thought for a moment and then said, "It is made out of Crisco and sugar."

That is kind of disgusting when you stop to think about it—those cakes were coated with a veneer of pure fat and sugar. Then I asked, "How long have you had these cakes on display?"

She told me, "They have been here *for the past five years.*" I just looked at her. What could I say?

Do you know why those cakes were kept under glass? It wasn't to preserve them—it was simply to keep the dust off the cakes so they would stay clean. Those cakes didn't need a preservation effort.

You can do the same thing with a tub of Crisco or any other partially hydrogenated oil. I challenge you to take a tub of Crisco, or any vegetable-shortening product, and set it on a shelf in your garage with the lid removed so its contents will be exposed to the open air. Believe me, it won't matter. You can leave it there for five, ten, fifteen or twenty years, and it still won't matter. Nothing will eat it. Sure, an insect may crawl in, get stuck and die there. But I assure you they won't eat it— they know better. God gave insects and the animal kingdom enough intrinsic knowledge to know better than to eat this synthetic stuff.

Anyone who has to use Crisco on a regular basis for cooking and baking purposes can tell you how hard it is to remove the stuff from their stove tops and from their hands and hair. Ask them what happens when the stuff lands on their clothes. It is almost impossible to remove from many fabrics. If you are really brave, talk to a plumber about what Crisco and similar products do to kitchen drains and plumbing in general. Ask them what it takes to actually remove these things from clogged drain pipes. The process may only begin with caustic pipe cleaners like Drano.

Now ask yourself, How is this stuff supposed to be removed from your arteries? You already know that drain cleaners cannot be put down your throat, so I guess that leaves the medical procedures of angioplasty and surgery—not very attractive alternatives, are they? I think you are getting my point. Margarine and other partially hydrogenated trans-fat products are some of the worst things that you can put into your system. As far as I am concerned, the stuff is as close to plastic as you can get without actually eating plastic.

Despite what you hear from the manufacturers and television ads, butter is actually better for you than margarine. No, I am not saying that butter is a health-food product, because it is not. However, butter—even with its high saturated-fat content—is healthier for your body than any trans-fat margarine product.

THERE IS AN ATTRACTIVE ALTERNATIVE

MANY PEOPLE FIND it very difficult to quit the margarine habit "cold turkey," so I have found an attractive alternative that lets you enjoy a spread on your bread without too much of a spread around your waist. One of the best alternatives is to use butter with equal parts of cold-pressed virgin olive oil and a little fresh garlic. You will have to keep it refrigerated of course, but at least you will have a viable alternative to margarine products.

A simple way to prepare this recipe is to allow the butter to warm to room temperature so that it acquires a soft texture. Then place it in a blender with an equal amount of olive oil. After the two ingredients have been blended together, put the mixture into the refrigerator until it hardens. You won't be able to taste the difference, but you will end up with a much healthier mix of monounsaturated fat and saturated fat. This blend is much easier to digest—and research has proven it a lot easier on your arteries—than a partially hydrogenated margarine product.

The best choice, of course, is to stop using butter and margarine products altogether in favor of modest amounts of straight virgin cold-pressed olive oil. Again, if you mix a little bit of garlic in with the oil, your healthy dressing will acquire a delicious flavor that can be basted on whole-grain breads and used as a dressing for salads. Remember that if your primary health goal is to lose weight, then you need to stay away from *all oils* as much as possible. Even the good oils are still liquid fat, so you don't want to use a lot of oil in your food or in your cooking. Of the calories in oil, 100 percent come from fat, so they should be avoided if you are trying to lose weight. (The only exceptions are the essential fatty acids previously mentioned. Your daily requirements for these essential nutrients can be supplied through daily supplementation with capsules of evening primrose oil, flaxseed oil and cod liver oil.)

MILLIONS OF
AMERICANS WILL SIT
DOWN FOR BREAKFAST,
LUNCH AND DINNER
TODAY AND EMPTY A
BLUE PACKET OF
ASPARTAME INTO THEIR
COFFEE OR TEA,
TOTALLY OBLIVIOUS
TO THE DANGERS . . .

Fourteen

THE BITTER FACTS ABOUT ASPARTAME AND DIET SODAS

ANOTHER OFFENDER ON the "Ten Foods You Should Never Eat" list is best known for its distinctive blue package and its brand names—burned into our psyche with a multimillion-dollar ad blitz. Its generic name is aspartame, but most people know it as NutraSweet and Equal. Millions of Americans will sit down for breakfast, lunch, and dinner today and empty a blue packet of aspartame into their coffee or tea, totally oblivious to the dangers...

Don't be fooled. The best-selling artificial sweetener in America wasn't the product of years of dedicated research by teams of researchers who were seeking a healthy nonsugar substitute for hard-pressed victims of diabetes, obesity or blood sugar problems. It was an accident, a clumsy laboratory slip-up that hit the big time faster than anyone could imagine.

James Schlatter, Ph. D., was conducting research for the G. D. Searle Company on a drug designed to treat ulcers. In December 1965, while Dr. Schlatter worked in the laboratory on his prospective anti-ulcer medication, he mixed a substance in a container with methanol (wood alcohol). Some of the substance accidentally spilled to the outside of the flask. When Dr. Schlatter picked up the flask, the substance rubbed onto his fingers. A few moments later when Dr. Schlatter licked his fingers to pick up a piece of paper, he reportedly noticed a very strong sweet taste. Dr. Schlatter soon discovered the sweetness had come from the contents of his experiment.[1] From this laboratory accident a legacy of deception has been forged against humanity. In this chapter you will find a full discussion of the deleterious effects of aspartame on the human body.

Under regular FDA guidelines, when a new chemical designed for human consumption is invented in the United States, it normally takes a long time to get from the laboratory to the kitchen table. Under most circumstances these chemicals are tested extensively on laboratory animals, and then tested on human subjects before they are ever allowed to be manufactured and sold for human use. If the chemicals are found to be reasonably safe ("reasonably safe" meaning that they are found to cause cancer in less than three in one million people), they are allowed to be marketed for human consumption.

Chemicals that are not shown to be safe for human use are not supposed to earn FDA approval. These products must go back to the laboratory for further research and development, which is a very costly venture for the manufacturer. If the chemical is found to be hazardous to one's health after it has been authorized for marketing, the chemicals are supposed to be pulled from the market, as was the case for Red Dye #19. If the product is not recalled, a warning label must be attached, as is the case for saccharine. NutraSweet, touted as the most tested product in the world, has managed to beat this system. Unknown to the general public, the company that manufactures aspartame has been accused of providing falsified test results to the FDA and even unethical deal making with prosecutors from the United States Attorney General's office. All the while, reports of adverse patient reactions including headaches, memory loss and seizures, and even confirmed death continue to mount while these reports are being kept from the general public.

UNHEEDED WARNINGS

INVESTIGATION INTO THE early stages of aspartame testing for human consumption reveals that serious questions regarding its safety began to surface as early as 1970. Nearly thirty years ago top researchers from Searle laboratories addressed their genuine concern over safety questions discovered while studying this chemical. Their initial concern revolved around the fact that they discovered a complete absence of legitimate study on the possible toxic effects aspartame could have on the human body. They also learned that no research was conducted on the possible toxic effects of the by-products of aspartame metabolism in the body.

For example, unknown to most NutraSweet consumers, aspartame breaks down in the body into its component chemicals, including methanol, aspartic acid, phenylalanine and a little known chemical called diketopiperazine (DKP).[2] Each of these component parts is in itself a known toxin. Apparently, this fact was not made completely clear by those who originally sought to gain aspartame's approval. David Baine, associate director of the U.S. General Accounting Office (GAO), stated that methyl alcohol was not even included in the initial description of aspartame provided by Searle when the company applied for FDA approval.

Methanol, also known as wood alcohol, has caused blindness in countless alcoholics. It is often used as a paint thinner and an industrial cleaner. When methanol is metabolized by the body, it is broken down into formaldehyde (yes, just like embalming fluid) and formic acid. *Steadman's Medical Dictionary* describes *methanol* as "a toxic, mobile liquid used as an industrial solvent, antifreeze and in chemical manufacture; ingestion may result in severe acidosis, visual impairment and other effects of the central nervous system."[3] The Environmental Protection Agency includes methanol in their Community Right to Know List, which is a list of toxic chemicals that must be clearly identified on manufacturers' labels when certain hazardous chemicals are used in a product. Amazingly, however, methanol is not mentioned on any of the labels of products containing aspartame.[4]

Effects in the body from human consumption of methanol include lethargy, fainting, headaches, nausea and vomiting, blindness, cough, breathing difficulties and other vision problems. Methanol has been shown to cause birth defects in developing fetuses, as well as other reproductive defects. According to *Sax's Dangerous Properties of Industrial Materials:*

> The main toxic effect [of methanol] is exerted upon the nervous system, particularly the optic nerve, and possibly the retinae, which can progress to permanent blindness. Once absorbed, methanol is only very slowly

eliminated. Coma resulting from massive exposures may last as long as two to four days. The products formed in the body by its oxidation are formaldehyde and formic acid, both of which are toxic. Because of its slow elimination, methanol should be regarded as a *cumulative* poison. Though single exposure to it may cause no harmful effect, daily exposure may result in the accumulation of sufficient methanol in the body to cause illness. Death from ingestion of less than 30 milliliters has been reported.[5]

To bring things into perspective, just one little blue packet of NutraSweet (1 gram) breaks down into 100 milligrams of methanol. Researchers have shown that a child who consumes 700 milligrams of aspartame (or less than three-fourths of one little blue packet) would be ingesting almost ten times the Environmental Protection Agency's (EPA) recommended daily limit of methanol consumption for a child.[6] The results can be worse if the product has been exposed to heat or left for a long time on the shelf, because these factors promote the breakdown of aspartame into its toxic components. Considering these facts, researchers are concerned that when high-consumption levels combine with aspartame's unstable shelf life, methanol can easily reach toxic levels in the systems of the millions of people who consume these products.[7]

DID ASPARTAME TRIGGER A NATIONAL EPIDEMIC OF BRAIN TUMORS?

DESPITE THESE HAZARDS Searle went forward with the process of receiving the FDA's approval for the use of aspartame as an artificial sweetener.[8] After only a year and a half, aspartame received an initial limited FDA approval for use in dry foods and chewing gum.[9] Objections by consumer watchdog groups were voiced immediately. James Turner, a consumer safety attorney, and Dr. John Olney, research psychiatrist at the Washington University School of Medicine, filed legal objections to aspartame's approval. The team resented documented evidence that animals fed the chemical during research conducted by Dr. Olney developed *brain tumors*. The health advocates demonstrated that aspartame ingestion could easily cause brain damage and mental retardation in humans. Turner and Olney requested that an immediate Public Board of Inquiry on the safety of aspartame be held by the FDA.[10]

In response to these objections and because it was evident that Searle had submitted false information on their animal research to the FDA in order to win approval, Commissioner Alexander

Schmidt of the FDA appointed a task force to investigate Searle's animal studies on aspartame. Six months later the FDA's task force report was in. The scathing report stated that some of Searle's research practices were too inappropriate even to be considered legitimate scientific research. The report went on to say that Searle's reports to the FDA were too unreliable to determine whether the product was safe for human consumption. Because of these findings, the FDA initially withheld approval of aspartame. However, these actions also delayed the Public Board of Inquiry requested by Turner and Olney.[11] Finally, in March 1976 the FDA's task force presented a completed report to Chairman Schmidt. The task force reported:

> At the heart of the FDA's regulatory process is its ability to rely upon the integrity of the basic safety data submitted by sponsors of regulated products. Our investigation clearly demonstrates that, in the G. D. Searle Company, we have no basis for such reliance now.... Some of our findings suggest an attitude of disregard for the FDA's mission of protection of the public health by selectively reporting the results of studies in a manner that allays the concerns of questions of an FDA reviewer.[12]

Because of these damaging findings, the FDA deepened its investigation of the research studies on aspartame.[13]

Another frightening correlation is the relationship of the introduction of NutraSweet to the American public and the surge in incidence of human brain tumors. In the *Journal of Advancement in Medicine,* scientist and researchers have cited that according to National Cancer Institute records, there has been a dramatic rise in the incidence of brain tumors in the United States beginning in 1985, just two years after NutraSweet became available in diet sodas. During that time the incidence of these brain tumors increased 600 percent! And the rise has continued every year since that time.

Researchers also point to aspartame in some cases of Alzheimer's disease. *On Call,* a medical society journal, draws attention to the amino acids in aspartame and their relation to the amino acids used as neurotransmitters in the brain. The article states that phenylalanine, aspartic acid, methanol and metabolites have been shown to "alter binding of excitatory amino acids to neuronal membranes and dysfunction of amino acid-derived neurotransmitters." The authors continue that "these findings raise concerns as to whether aspartame might initiate or aggravate Alzheimer's disease."[14]

The situation began to look grim for the G. D. Searle Company and to any further FDA approval of their product. In January 1977, U.S. Attorney Sam Skinner was contacted by the Chief Counsel of the FDA, Richard Merrill. Chief Counsel Merrill requested that a grand jury be convened to investigate Searle for "violations of the Federal Food, Drug and Cosmetic Act...and the False Reports to the Government Act...for their willful and knowing failure to make reports to the Food and Drug Administration...and for concealing material facts and making false statements in reports of animal studies conducted to establish the safety of [aspartame]." FDA Chief Counsel Merrill specifically cited two of Searle's studies.

One study was on the effects of aspartame on monkeys while the other examined aspartame toxicity in hamsters. In the instance of the primate study, the FDA task force discovered that some of the monkeys fed aspartame suffered seizures, a fact that was never reported to the FDA when Searle applied for the approval of aspartame. In what many could consider an attempt to cover up the true cause of the seizures, researchers disposed of the primates without ever completing autopsies to determine the true cause of this erratic brain activity.[15]

DECEPTION AND COVER-UP?

IN THIS INVESTIGATION, Searle was represented by a prestigious and powerful Chicago law firm,

Sidley and Austin. Just two weeks after Merrill's letter was sent to Skinner, the office of Sidley and Austin contacted U.S. Attorney Skinner and requested a private meeting prior to the grand jury hearing.[16] Seven days after their private meeting, Sidley and Austin offered Skinner a high-paying position within their law firm.[17] It is important to note here that the statute of limitations for prosecution against the G. D. Searle Company for their alleged violations was rapidly drawing near.[18] Without Skinner's immediate action, any legal avenues of prosecution against Searle would be lost forever. U.S. Attorney Skinner was personally reminded by the Justice Department of the urgent need to proceed with the grand jury investigation due to the statute of limitations.[19] Unfortunately, without going forward with the investigation, Skinner left his post with the U.S. Attorney General's office on July 1, 1977, and joined the law office of Sidley and Austin, not leaving sufficient time for his successor to launch the grand jury investigation before it was too late.[20]

In August 1977, another team of FDA investigators, under the direction of Jerome Bressler, investigated Searle's research practices on the safety of aspartame and published the Bressler Report. This report cited that during one Searle animal research program on the safety of aspartame, which was never reported to the FDA, ninety-eight of the one hundred ninety-six animals died during the study. That is 50 percent! The FDA investigators found that rather than try to discover what killed these lab animals immediately, Searle researchers did not perform autopsies until in some instances *over one full year* after the animals' deaths. Obviously, if the company had any interest in your safety, they would have immediately searched for a complete explanation.

Food and Drug Administration investigators also found blatant discrepancies between the pathology records they were provided and those maintained in the laboratory. The number of reported brain lesions and tumors found during the autopsies in the animals fed aspartame were markedly different from reports submitted by Searle to the FDA and those found in the research laboratory.

Several other inconsistencies in Searle's reporting were also discovered. In one instance, a specific rat was reported to be alive for a number of days, then the rat died. Later, however, the *same rat* in the *same study* was reported to be alive again, only to die a second time. At the very least, this is evidence of sloppy research and, arguably, complete fraud. The FDA investigators also discovered cases of tumors, uterine growths and ovarian growths that were documented on laboratory-held reports, but were not noted in Searle's reports to the FDA.

When the FDA's Center for Food Investigations later conducted research on aspartame, they found that uterine polyps or growths occurred in at least 15 percent of the lab animals in their study (a fact consistent with the reports found in Searle's labs that were withheld from the FDA).[21]

The FDA investigation and the Bressler Report were under the oversight of the FDA Bureau of Foods, chaired by H. R. Roberts, who was the highest-ranking recipient of the report. Completely disregarding the obvious discrepancies outlined in the Bressler Report, Roberts announced that he would consider Searle's research as acceptable and apparently authentic for the FDA. In this decision, considered unconscionable by many, Roberts overrode the discoveries and recommendations of the Bressler Report and recommended further FDA approval of the controversial chemical. Because of his position in the FDA, this meant that Roberts' decision would largely go unchallenged. However, in an apparent conflict of interest, H. R. Roberts subsequently left the FDA and became the vice president of the U.S. National Soft Drink Association.[22] The benefits that the approval of aspartame for use in carbonated beverages would offer to the soft drink industry made its approval a *multibillion-dollar* prospect.

Continuing Controversy

In June 1979, five years after Olney's and Turner's request, the FDA finally established the Public Board of Inquiry (PBI). The stated purpose of this board was to investigate and rule on safety issues surrounding NutraSweet.[23] It was not until January 1980 that the PBI finally began actually holding its hearings. However, the evidence against aspartame was so conclusive that the PBI recommended to the FDA that NutraSweet should not be approved until further investigations had been conducted on the incidence of brain tumors in animals. The FDA-organized board further reported that there was no decisive evidence that aspartame was at all safe as a food additive.[24]

In spite of further studies recommending that NutraSweet not be approved as a food additive for human consumption, the legitimate concerns and questions raised by the PBI and FDA scientists were largely ignored by the hierarchy of the FDA. By October 1981 aspartame had been approved for use as a table-top sweetener, in tablets, cold breakfast cereals, dry bases for beverages, instant coffee and tea, gelatins, puddings, fillings, dairy-product-analog toppings and as a flavor enhancer for chewing gum. Most alarming of these approved uses are those products that are served hot, like hot chocolate, coffee and tea, because heat speeds the breakdown of aspartame.[25] Going forward with its efforts to expand the market of NutraSweet worldwide, Searle petitioned the FDA to approve aspartame for use as a sweetener in carbonated beverage syrup bases and other liquids.[26]

However, at this time even the National Soft Drink Association (NSDA) was not comfortable with Searle's request. In July 1983, the NSDA urged the FDA to delay approval of aspartame for carbonated beverages pending further testing because temperature had been shown to speed the breakdown of aspartame. The NSDA's concern was due to the fact that when their products were shipped or stored, it was very difficult to regulate their temperature. On hot summer days, a bottle of beverage in the back of a closed semitrailer sitting in the sun can become *extremely* hot. The FDA responded that they were aware of the problem with temperature and aspartame, but that the FDA believed proper shipping and marketing procedures would "solve" the problems.[27]

In spite of these objections, on July 8, 1983, NutraSweet was approved for use in carbonated beverages and carbonated beverage-syrup bases by acting commissioner of the FDA, Mark Novitch. Approval was granted despite the knowledge that when aspartame-sweetened beverages are stored for as little as *eight weeks* even at reasonably cool temperatures below 68 degrees Fahrenheit, up to

20 percent of the aspartame would be broken down to its basic elements. (The "lost" aspartame degrades to DKP, methanol [methyl alcohol], aspartic acid and phenylalanine.[28]) According to the 1985 Congressional Record, when aspartame-laced products are stored or heated above 85 degrees for a period as short as a few weeks (such as when products are produced, stored, shipped to the marketplace, stored on shelves, purchased by consumers and left in the pantry or garage until desired), *absolutely no aspartame is left in the beverage, only its by-products.*[29]

CONCERNS THAT WON'T GO AWAY

CONCERNS OVER THE safety of aspartame use continued to grow. In the July 1984 issue of *Common Cause* magazine, Florence Graves, editor and vice president of publications, writes:

> NutraSweet has been touted as the most tested food additive in history, but our investigation reveals such serious flaws in the government's approval of NutraSweet that Congress should begin its own investigation immediately.[30]

By this time, the Center for Disease Control (CDC) had received almost six hundred reported cases of adverse health complaints from patients after ingesting aspartame, but because of the overwhelming number, CDC had only been able to review two hundred thirteen of the reports. Patients ranged from four-month-old children to seventy-seven-year-old senior citizens. More than 25 percent reported experiencing similar ailments each time they consumed a product containing aspartame. Symptoms varied; however, many reported disorientation, hyperactivity, extreme numbness, excitability, memory loss, seizures, suicidal tendencies and severe mood swings.

In a special report, the Center for Disease Control recommended that future aspartame research focus on the neurological, emotional and human behavior problems manifested in their patients' complaints.[31] Ironically, in complete conflict with his own organization's report, Frederick L. Trowbridge, an executive for the CDC, added an unsolicited appendix to the report. In his annex, Trowbridge argued that "currently available information based on data with limitations as described in the report, indicated a wide variety of complaints that are generally of a mild nature. Although it may be that certain individuals have an unusual sensitivity to the product, these data do not provide evidence for the existence of serious, widespread, adverse health consequences to the use of aspartame."[32] How can reports of patient problems such as aggressive behavior, disorientation, hyperactivity, extreme numbness, excitability, memory loss, loss of depth perception, liver impairment, cardiac arrest, seizures, suicidal tendencies and severe mood swings be considered "of a mild nature"?

It is obvious that genuine concern for our well-being is not everyone's priority. I shudder to think what motivates someone to ignore the plight of honest citizens who suffer genuine health problems when they ingest a product supposedly harmless to them. The irregularities, conflicts of interest and apparent fraud have somehow been largely ignored by the mainstream news media. Even *Editor and Publisher Magazine*, a periodical for journalists, in the July 13, 1985, issue reported "The Food and Drug Administration NutraSweet cover-up" as one of the most under-reported stories of the year.[33]

WIDER APPROVAL IN THE FACE OF WIDER CONCERNS

IN 1986, GEORGE R. Verrilli, M.D., and Anne Marie Mueser published a book for expectant mothers titled *While Waiting: A Prenatal Guidebook*. In this book Dr. Verrilli and Ms. Mueser raised concern over the effects aspartame could have on babies growing in the womb. The team wrote that "aspartame is suspected of causing brain damage in sensitive individuals. A fetus may be at risk for these effects...some researchers have suggested that high doses of aspartame may be associated with problems ranging from dizziness and subtle brain changes to mental retardation."[34]

As time progressed, the justification for public concern continued to intensify. On February 3, 1986, Senator Howard Metzenbaum released documents from a congressional investigation of aspartame and the G. D. Searle Company. In these documents, the senator discovered that during at least one Searle research project on primates, every monkey that received either medium or large doses of NutraSweet suffered debilitating seizures. This was just another fact withheld from the FDA,[35] yet the product remains on the market. On July 17, 1986, consumer attorney James Turner filed a petition on behalf of the Consumer Nutrition Institute, seeking to force the FDA to reconsider its regulations regarding safe use of aspartame and to change the current regulations.[36] Three months later, in a legal maneuver, Turner filed a citizen's petition over aspartame, citing that use of the chemical inherently had hazards of seizures and possible eye damage.[37] Without having the evidence of NutraSweet's adverse reactions presented for any evaluation, the FDA denied the petitions.[38] Only one week later, ever pressing in on its efforts, aspartame was approved by the FDA for use in concentrated fruit juices and fruit flavored drinks, frozen popsicles, breath mints and teas.[39]

The very next month the FDA declared aspartame, provided labeling met certain specifications, as safe for use as an inactive ingredient. By calling aspartame "inactive," the FDA completely disregarded all the evidence that has demonstrated the toxic effects of aspartame and the apparent cover-up conducted by researchers.[40] In a bizarre contradiction, the same month that the FDA labeled aspartame as "an inactive ingredient," the FDA published a list of seventy-three adverse symptoms associated with aspartame use, which included four deaths attributed to its use. Two weeks later, in January 1987, an FDA quarterly report on the adverse reactions associated with aspartame was released. This report cited that the FDA had received *3,133 consumer complaints* of adverse reactions associated with aspartame use. The FDA publication cited that the majority of the complaints referred to neurological symptoms, including severe headache, dizziness, numbness and loss of memory.[41]

By the beginning of 1988, almost five hundred products directly marketed to American consumers contained the potentially lethal chemical.[42] Another FDA quarterly report on adverse reactions associated with aspartame was released on October 1, 1988. This report stated that the FDA had received over 4,200 consumer complaints against aspartame ingestion. As with previous information of the hazards associated with the use of this chemical, this report did not generate any action to truly evaluate aspartame safety risks by the government office designed to protect your health.[43]

"A CRIME AGAINST HUMANITY"

NUMEROUS SPECIALISTS IN the health field have spoken out against aspartame use. One of these is Woodrow Monte, R.D., Ph.D., director of the Arizona State University Food Sciences and Nutrition Laboratory. When I spoke with Dr. Monte in December 1994, he expressed his vehement objection to the methanol content of aspartame, calling aspartame a "crime against humanity." Monte argued that:

> Humans are a hundred times more sensitive to methanol than are animals. This means when studies of the effects of aspartame on animals are compared for human use, the adverse effects must be multiplied one hundred times. When a person ingests aspartame, it breaks down into methanol within one hour of ingestion. Methanol is formed as soon as aspartame is added into a solution and continues to form the longer it is in solution.[44]

Dr. Monte also expressed concern over the widespread use of NutraSweet in America because heat speeds the breakdown of aspartame into methanol. According to Dr. Monte, who has conducted countless hours of research and experimentation of this chemical, if aspartame is added to a hot beverage, say hot chocolate, coffee or tea at 80 degrees Celsius (145 degrees Fahrenheit), *one half of the amount of aspartame originally added breaks down into methanol in less than ten minutes.*[45]

Dr. Monte is very concerned about the FDA's 1993 approval for the use of aspartame in baked goods and other heated products, not to mention products like flavored coffees and hot chocolates, which have been on the market for several years now. Reminding me that aspartame began its existence as a product for a prescription medication, Dr. Monte stated that he believes aspartame was mislabeled from the beginning. "Aspartame is a drug, not a food additive," he informed me. "One hundred million people, from pregnant women to little babies to the elderly, are consuming this stuff in megadoses. This product is being consumed more than it ever would if it were labeled as a drug, as it was originally intended to be."

While Dr. Ralph Walton was chief of psychiatry at New York's Jamestown Hospital, he treated a fifty-four-year-old female who had suffered a grand mal seizure with no prior history of seizure activity. Following the seizure, the patient's behavior became bizarre and uncharacteristic. Dr. Walton could find no clinical reason for the patient's mental status change, and he began to question her on any changes she may have experienced in her daily lifestyle. It appeared that the woman generally drank about a gallon of sugar-sweetened tea daily for years. However, shortly before her seizure she had replaced the sugar in her tea with NutraSweet in order to lose some weight.

Dr. Walton advised his patient to refrain from using the chemical product, and within a very short period of time she became like her old self again. Today, Dr. Walton does not trust the research Searle produced to win FDA approval. The doctor stated, "I know it causes seizures. I'm convinced also that it definitely causes behavioral changes. I'm very angry that this substance is on the market. I personally question the reliability and validity of any studies funded by the NutraSweet Company."[46]

An internal medicine physician practicing in the state of Florida, Dr. H. J. Roberts, produced a work reporting several case studies of individuals who had been adversely affected by consuming aspartame. Dr. Roberts described one horrible incident where a college honor student was irreversibly debilitated due to destruction left in the wake of aspartame use. In this case history, Dr. Roberts told the story of how this eighteen-year-old college student sought his treatment in 1986 because of "profound intellectual deterioration." According to Dr. Roberts, the patient was previously an outstanding student at a major university, a skilled typist and pianist. However, her skills had rapidly declined, and she had suffered a loss of twenty IQ points by the time of her first visit to his office. She went to the doctor complaining of severe headaches, inability to sleep restfully, suicidal depression and an itching in the genital region. She also suffered a burning sensation when she urinated, a dramatic change in her personality, stomach pain and nausea. The female patient had stopped having monthly periods and experienced an ironic fifteen-pound weight gain while dieting.

Dr. Roberts immediately began a battery of extensive physical, blood and neurological tests on the woman. Following this exhaustive array of tests, the doctor could not find any patterns consistent with a known form of organic brain problem or schizophrenia. The patient's problems fit no known scenario or normal pattern of disease, which at first baffled Dr. Roberts. Upon observing the patient, Dr. Roberts noted that she became drowsy after she drank a diet soda with aspartame. Upon investigation, the patient revealed that she consumed a large quantity of diet soda, and had done so for a period of time.

At that point the physician advised his patient to avoid aspartame products completely. Following abstinence from NutraSweet-laced products, the patient was also advised to follow a diet rich in complex carbohydrates and with few refined sugars to prevent fluctuations in her blood glucose. According to Dr. Roberts, avoidance of aspartame relieved her symptoms, but the apparent brain damage remained. Ultimately, this patient had to be placed in a halfway-type program for the mentally challenged.[47]

ALARMING AIRLINE RESEARCH ABOUT ASPARTAME

IN AUGUST 1987, Mary Stoddard organized the Aspartame Consumer Safety Network to help those who were afflicted with aspartame-sensitivity problems.[48] Ms. Stoddard's efforts were the direct result of her personal debilitating experience after consuming products made with NutraSweet. When Stoddard's health began to decline in 1984 after she began a diet, she began to experience dozens of strange symptoms that she had never felt before, including blurred vision, depression, ringing in her ears, muscle tremors, weakness in her arms and legs with cramping of those muscles, a nervous-type twitch in her body, congested ears, sores on her skin, sinus congestion, joint pains and even a loss in her hearing.

Eventually, Mary Stoddard began to suspect that the diet products she consumed containing aspartame were at the root of her health problems. On that hunch she decided to eliminate NutraSweet from her diet completely, and she reported that she began to feel better immediately. Unfortunately, it took six months for all of her symptoms to completely recede. During her recovery, Ms. Stoddard unknowingly ate a product that used aspartame as a sweetener. She reported that her symptoms returned, proving to her that aspartame was at the root of her troubles.

Currently Ms. Stoddard focuses much of her attention on pilots and the aviation industry in general. "I shudder to think of what would happen if just one of our airline pilots suffered a seizure while in the cockpit," Ms. Stoddard stated. "I am receiving literally hundreds of calls from pilots who have either lost their flight status due to symptoms, especially seizures, from consuming NutraSweet, or who have experienced severe reactions but have been able to cover up their problems from FAA physicians. Countless pilots have told me personally of nearly disastrous events that occurred while flying under the influence of aspartame."

It appears that numerous pilots have experienced seizures and other bizarre health changes as a result of consuming beverages sweetened with Nutra-Sweet. Once a pilot has any type of a seizure, he or she is usually grounded for life, and their career is over. The U.S. military has begun to express genuine concern over the issue of NutraSweet and its pilots. Scientists at the U.S. Armed Forces Institute of Pathology (AFIP) have examined the research and papers written on NutraSweet since 1970 and warn that consuming aspartame may lead to blood pressure instability and disturbances in visual perception. A spokesperson for AFIP expressed grave concern for pilots. When a pilot experiences any difficulties with visual perception while in the cockpit, much less seizures, the results could be a national tragedy.[49] The official Air Force safety magazine, *Flying Safety,* and the Navy's *Navy Physiology* have both published warnings to their pilots to refrain from using the chemical.

Perhaps one of the most frightening circumstantial events surrounding aspartame and flight safety came from the voice recorder on board USAir Flight 427, which crashed near Pittsburgh International Airport on September 8, 1994, killing all one hundred thirty-two people on board. Conversation in the cockpit was quite normal, until the pilot, Capt. Peter Germano, consumed a national-brand diet soft drink just ten minutes before the crash. Other pilots have reported having seizures while in flight following their use of diet sodas, narrowly escaping the same fate. We are only left to speculate what role aspartame played in this tragic event, if any. However, according to FAA investigators, the aircraft itself was not to blame in the crash.

STILL SITTING ON STORE SHELVES

THE YEARS THAT have followed the release of this toxic substance on the American population have been met with literally thousands of consumer complaints of adverse heath effects associated with consumption of products containing aspartame. In February 1994, the Department of Health and Human Services Report on Adverse Reactions Attributed to Aspartame for 1993, reported 6,888 consumer complaints, including 649 reported by the Centers for Disease Control, and another 1,305 reported by the FDA. Currently, *aspartame accounts for over 75 percent of all the complaints in the Adverse Reaction Monitoring System.* Yet, the use of this product grows every day, and your FDA does nothing.

With all the controversy aspartame and its marketed product, NutraSweet, have generated, I am truly startled that it has remained on our store shelves. I am very dismayed that those government agencies we have trusted to protect us have done so little. But armed with this knowledge, there is no reason why you should choose to let it remain in your diet!

This completes another of the "Foods You Should Never Eat." I call high-fat luncheon meat, shellfish, margarine and aspartame the "Kevorkian Four" in honor of America's premiere suicide doctor. My reasoning should be obvious—if you eat these foods on a regular basis, then you are committed to "suicide on the installment plan." Avoid these foods at all costs.

OLESTRA TAKES THE THEME OF "FOOLING MOTHER NATURE" TO AN ENTIRELY NEW LEVEL.

Fifteen

HOLD THE OLESTRA
AND LIVE LONGER

THERE IS A new thorn in the FDA's side, a fake fat that really had its beginning as a trial drug meant to control cholesterol. When the "drug" didn't perform very well, Proctor & Gamble withdrew its application for drug approval and applied for approval of its hybrid fake fat as a food additive. This upstart newcomer seems to have created an even bigger storm of complaints than aspartame!

Years ago, one of the leading brand-name margarines ran a series of television and magazine ads based on the theme, "It's not polite to fool Mother Nature..." The intent of the ad was to say that this brand of margarine tasted so much like butter "that even Mother Nature was fooled." Nature wasn't fooled then, and it's not fooled now. The human body has quickly caught on to a new pretender in the snack sections of our grocery stores.

Olestra takes the theme of "fooling Mother Nature" to an entirely new level. Proctor & Gamble's chemists created this "nonabsorbable cooking oil" by combining vegetable oil and sucrose (sugar) to produce a molecule with physical characteristics similar to fat/triglyceride. The alleged benefit is that this "cooking oil" adds no fat or calories to the diet. In a way, the manufacturer's claims are true, but the way this product "delivers" on that promise is anything but pleasant or desirable.

This Fake Fat Just "Passes Through"

Proctor & Gamble's literature says, "While triglyceride consists of a glycerol core with three fatty acids attached, olestra is composed of a sucrose core with six to eight fatty acid chains attached. This tight structural configuration prevents olestra from being metabolized by digestive enzymes or colonic microflora."[1] In other words, olestra isn't broken down or absorbed in the gastrointestinal (GI) tract. It literally passes through the GI tract unchanged! The company literature lightly acknowledges the fact that consumers have experienced some problems, but quickly moves into a defensive posture. I wonder why? Proctor & Gamble says:

Some people who eat snacks made with olestra may notice digestive changes, such as softer stools. These changes are similar to those experienced after eating poorly absorbed foods such as high-fiber bran. Similarly, whether patients notice this effect may depend upon the interactions they normally experience between changes in their diets and their bowel movements. This should not be confused with diarrhea.[2]

In the same document, Proctor & Gamble admitted that their wonder drug/fake fat had what they term "an OIT" problem. Once you realize what it is, you will wonder what makes people want to try this product in the first place. However, I do strongly endorse the final comment in this paragraph as the ultimate solution to the olestra problem:

Droplets of oil in the toilet water (OIT) can occur when olestra separates from the fecal matrix upon dispersion in the toilet water...Consumers who eat large enough quantities of olestra snacks that they observe OIT should be reassured that this effect is not a result of lipid malabsorption and the change in stool, if bothersome, will resolve when they decrease or stop consumption of olestra snacks.[3]

Evidently there are thousands of dissatisfied customers who would disagree with Proctor & Gamble. According to a news release issued in December 1998 by a nonprofit health group called the Center for Science in the Public Interest (CSPI), fifteen thousand customers had already filed complaints about olestra with Proctor & Gamble and CSPI.

Virtually all of the consumers who took the trouble to file a complaint said they experienced problems ranging from gas to bloody stools to cramps so severe that they had to go to the emergency room. The symptoms surfaced after each victim ate Wow snack chips (a special version of five or more preexisting chip products marketed by Frito-Lay) or Fat-Free Pringles (a product of Proctor & Gamble). Both of these product lines are advertised as being fat-free because they are made using olestra.

AS MANY AS 60 PERCENT MAY BE AFFECTED

THE FIFTEEN THOUSAND reported cases of olestra poisoning may only be the tip of the iceburg. Typically, only a tiny fraction of the people victimized by products ever contact the manufacturing company or a health agency. One study showed that as many as 60 percent may be affected if they eat a few ounces of Olean chips every day for several weeks. Other studies involving less frequent consumption find that much smaller percentages are affected.[4]

CSPI reported that more than one hundred people in the most recent group of complaints suffered such serious symptoms after eating small amounts of these chips that they *sought medical attention.* Forty of them *went to hospital emergency rooms,* where several were treated for dehydration. In some cases, doctors actually labeled olestra as the specific cause of the symptoms in their reports.

In a national news release issued by CSPI, victims reported experiencing side effects after eating chips prepared with olestra that ranged from mild inconvenience to serious safety risks: "Olestra made some people soil their clothing at work or school, ruin their vacations, miss work, leave young children unattended and vomit while driving. Two flight attendants and a military pilot said olestra prevented them from flying."[5]

Proctor & Gamble likes to say that Olean makes snacks "a little healthier." Frito-Lay's powerful marketing machine wants everyone to know that its Wow line of chips is "safe for everyone." Evidently, not everyone is buying it. CSPI reported that *The New England Journal of Medicine* has refused to run any more deceptive Olean ads. The Council of Better Business Bureaus also found that certain Olean ads were misleading because they implied that olestra is a natural substance and that it looks like an ordinary vegetable oil.

WOW! NINE TEASPOONS OF OLESTRA PER BAG!

OLEAN'S DOGGED ADVERSARY, CSPI, agrees that Olean's ads and labeling are deceptive. The non-profit health advocacy group filed a petition with the FDA urging that it not allow products made with Olean to be called "fat free." To prove its point, representatives displayed test tubes filled with *nine teaspoons of fake fat* extracted from *a single 5.5-ounce bag of Wow potato chips made with Olean!*

The FDA also received letters from Guiltless Gourmet and other makers of genuinely "fat-free" baked chips complaining that Proctor & Gamble's claim that Olean products are "fat free" is misleading and unfair.[6] When you think about those nine teaspoons of indigestible fat oozing out of a bag of "fat-free" chips, it is easy to understand why Guiltless Gourmet is unhappy.

Proctor & Gamble (and the line of eager food producers planning to use Olean to make "fat-free" foods and food products) probably hoped all of the furor would die down once olestra received its FDA approval. They were wrong. Even more opponents came out of the woodwork as the company neared a crucial FDA reevaluation of olestra's safety in 1998.

Dr. Walter Willett, chairman of the nutrition department at the Harvard School of Public Health, released a letter from fourteen prominent professors at Harvard, New York University, University of California at Berkeley and other institutions urging the FDA's Food Advisory Committee to recommend that olestra's approval be revoked. Opponents also included more than one hundred medical doctors, the former chief of nutrition at the United States Department of Agriculture and a top researcher at the National Cancer Institute. The American Public Health Association, The Lighthouse and the National Association for Visually Handicapped also have opposed olestra.[7]

WHO IS RAISING WHAT RHETORIC?

ONCE AGAIN, THE FDA turned a deaf ear to expert witnesses and wholeheartedly endorsed—or should I say *embraced*—Proctor & Gamble's fake-fat substitute, olestra. Two days before the FDA panel decision, Frito-Lay Chairman Steven Reinemund published an open letter in *The New York Times,* praising the safety of his company's products made with Olean in light of what he called "raised rhetoric" from the Center for Science in the Public Interest (CSPI). Frito-Lay said its Wow chips made with Olean are "the biggest new food and beverage product in this decade."[8] It sounds like Mr. Reinemund raised some rhetoric of his own.

When CSPI held a news conference in June 1988 on the dangers of olestra, several consumer-victims stepped forward voluntarily to warn others about the dangers of olestra. They didn't care about all of the "new studies" pouring out of Proctor & Gamble headquarters claiming that olestra doesn't do what *its own studies* proves it does. The victims didn't need manufacturer's studies to know this much: Olestra made them sick.

ONE VICTIM CALLED OLESTRA THE "FAKE FAT FROM HELL"

REGINA McGRATH, OF Hannastown, Pennsylvania, told reporters that she ate about twelve Doritos Nacho Cheese chips at lunch. "An hour later, I experienced such severe stomach pains that I went to the emergency room, where I was given intra-venous morphine. I was once in labor for twenty-one hours—*this pain was worse.*" Her final words may well sum up my point in this chapter. She said, "My doctor said that Olean was the cul-prit. *It hit me like the fake fat from hell.*"[9]

Claire Milford, a registered nurse from Indianapolis, experienced yellow stools, severe cramps and other symptoms the day after she ate

Proctor & Gamble's Wow chips. She went to the hospital where the doctor attributed the problem to olestra after not finding any other cause.[10]

Terri Crowder, a college student from Clinton, Maryland, said, "I suffered watery diarrhea and severe, almost debilitating, cramps several hours after eating about an ounce of Wow Ruffles potato chips. I had to go to bathroom numerous times during the night, at work and in classes."[11]

Dozens of Indiana residents who said they were affected by olestra gathered together in Indianapolis and marched to the Indiana State Department of Health to urge the department to "warn Hoosiers that olestra could cause great suffering in people of all ages." Bonnie Ross, a registered dietician from Indianapolis, is quoted as saying, "I am very concerned about the short- and long-term health risks associated with olestra. Many of my patients who tried olestra snacks suffered cramps and diarrhea. It seems unconscionable to allow a chemical like olestra to get into our food supply. The *only* benefit I can see from olestra is big-time profits for Proctor & Gamble."[12]

OLESTRA ROBS THE BODY OF CAROTENOIDS

PERHAPS THE MOST dangerous aspect of the olestra issue is its ability to absorb (or steal) crucial nutrients and antioxidants bound to natural fats while it "passes through" the human digestive system. Dr. Willett of the Harvard School of Public Health put it this way:

> Olestra actually has negative nutritional value because it prevents the body from absorbing carotenoids. Because of evidence that carotenoids protect against chronic diseases, long-term use of olestra in snack foods is likely to cause thousands of cases of cancer and heart disease each year.[13]

The *Medical Sciences Bulletin,* published by Pharmaceutical Information Associates, Ltd., issued a bulletin notifying its readers that the FDA had approved olestra as a "fat-free fat." However, the article had some interesting perspectives that weren't all that positive. It said, in part:

> Unfortunately, olestra does more than just pass silently through the intestines—it also picks up fat-soluble nutrients, including beta carotene and a host of other carotenoids and vitamins A, D, E and K. Studies have shown that *eating even a small snack bag of olestra-fried potato chips can reduce blood levels of beta carotene by 60 percent.* Since beta carotene deficiency is associated with cancer, heart dis-

ease and macular degeneration, *olestra may theoretically increase the risks of these diseases.* Snagging other fat-soluble vitamins could also lead to health problems. Vitamin D is involved in calcium metabolism, vitamin K in blood clotting and vitamin A (from the diet or produced from beta carotene) in immune function and vision, while the antioxidant vitamin E is thought to protect against cancer and heart disease.

In addition to vitamin deficiency, olestra can cause diarrhea and anal leakage (uncontrolled greasy seepage). P&G has reformulated the product to reduce the anal leakage and plans to fortify olestra-containing processed snack foods with extra vitamins. However, many scientists doubt that fortification will do any more than *fortify the greasy seepage* [italics mine].[14]

FDA: Who Cares About Carotenoids?

It is interesting to me that the FDA, in its official approval documents and press release announcing olestra's approval, acknowledged the problems I italicized in the excerpt above, but actually dismissed the entire beta carotene vitamin group as unimportant! An FDA news release said:

In addition to inhibiting the absorption of essential vitamins, olestra reduces the absorption of some carotenoids—nutrients found in carrots, sweet potatoes, green leaf vegetables and some animal tissue. The company's post-marketing monitoring of olestra consumption levels and additional studies will provide FDA with further information about olestra's effects on the absorption of carotenoids. *The role of carotenoids in human health is not fully understood* [italics mine]. FDA will continue to monitor all available scientific research on the role of carotenoids in human health.[15]

That single phrase, "The role of carotenoids in human health is not fully understood," describes how the FDA completely dismissed the importance of carotenoids in the human diet and olestra's dangerous ability to steal them from the very foods we eat.

This is especially odd when you consider what other more nutrition- and consumer-conscious departments in Washington, D.C., have to say about carotenoids. Evidently, the FDA (the "left hand" of the U.S. Government in this analogy) doesn't know what the "right hand" is doing.

Proctor & Gamble commissioned two eight-week clinical studies using 8 grams of olestra per day, the lowest level of the substance ever tested. After the test subjects ate the equivalent of *only sixteen potato chips* containing olestra, the studies revealed that olestra caused dramatic depletion of fat-soluble vitamins *in just two weeks!*

According to CSPI, the research studies also measured total serum carotenoids, alpha-carotene, beta carotene, lutein and lycopene. Olestra caused significant declines in all carotenoids monitored. Total serum carotenoids declined sharply by the fourteenth day of olestra consumption and was down by 50 to 60 percent by the end of the studies. A dosage of 32 grams per day of olestra (or about sixty-four olestra-saturated potato chips) reduced total serum carotenoids by 70 percent over the eight weeks.[16] A four-week study conducted in Holland demonstrated that olestra-like chemicals significantly lower beta carotene levels when you eat the equivalent of only *six olestra-saturated potato chips per day!*[17]

This problem can quickly spiral out of control if people include olestra products like fat-free potato chips, tortilla chips, fat-free Ritz crackers or fat-free Wheat Thins with two or more meals per day. The olestra in these products may increase risks of major disease and other health problems by reducing the body's ability to absorb vital beta carotene and fat-soluble vitamins from their food and dietary supplements.

Surgeon General:
We Care About Carotenoids!

AS YOU HAVE seen throughout this book in repeated references, cancer experts are urging us to eat much greater quantities of vegetables and fruits, in part because of their carotenoids and other phytochemicals. Beta carotene and other carotenoids have clearly been shown to reduce cancer incidence in animals exposed to carcinogens.[18] Diets rich in carotenoid-rich fruits and vegetables have been linked to lower risks of cancers of the lung, esophagus, pharynx, mouth, stomach, colon, rectum and bladder. *Low levels* of beta carotene in the blood, in particular, have been associated with high rates of stomach and lung cancer.[19]

When the Department of Health and Human Services issued the Surgeon General's Report on Nutrition and Health in 1988, the Surgeon General stated something the FDA evidently missed in their rush to approve olestra as the fake fat of choice for Americans:

> Epidemiological studies provide suggestive evidence that consumption of foods containing carotenoids, including the beta carotene precursor of vitamin A, protects against development of epithelial cell cancers such as those of the oral cavity, bladder, or

lung. These studies have generally shown *lower rates of cancer* among individuals consuming the highest overall levels of vitamin A, carotenoids or fruits and vegetables.[20]

The National Research Council echoed the sentiments of the Surgeon General in its 1989 report, "Diet and Health," when it stated, "[T]here is strong evidence that a *low intake of carotenoids, which are present in green and yellow vegetables, contributes to an increased risk of lung cancer.*"[21]

FDA's Approval of Olestra Defies Logic

THE CENTER FOR Science in the Public Interest noted that in January 1996, only three weeks before the FDA approved olestra, the FDA's "sister" agency under the U.S. Department of Health and Human Services urged people to consume carotenoid-rich fruits and vegetables because of their likely role in preventing cancer and other chronic diseases as part of its annual "Dietary Guidelines for Americans" edition, the primer of the nation's basic nutrition policies. The CSPI summarized the carotenoids issue as well as anyone could:

While there is not yet conclusive proof that carotenoids reduce cancer risk, to approve a major new additive that would significantly reduce levels of carotenoids (and possibly other fat-soluble phytochemicals) defies logic. It is a remarkable case of governmental ineptitude to have one agency of the Department of Health and Human Services, the National Cancer Institute, encouraging consumers to eat more carotenoid-rich fruits and vegetables, while another agency, the FDA, approves a food additive that depletes the body of potentially beneficial substances in those foods.[22]

Let me share a final irony to end this chapter on a lighter note. The FDA is careful to maintain separate food-safety regulations for animals. It gladly allows human snack foods made with Olean to be called "fat-free," presumably because without the deceptive labeling, human consumers would be unable to purchase and consume the product without worrying about the serious consequences that are indeed awaiting them.

The best "olestra quote" of all may belong to Dr. Tim Byers, a professor of preventive medicine at the University of Colorado Health Services Center, who commented on olestra's effects on carotenoids, saying, "Olestra-containing products should come with a warning label stating: 'Do not eat this product with food.'"[23]

I hope I've made my point about Olean or any other olestra-like products that may emerge. Just say, "Hold the Olean." You will definitely live longer and happier. There are better ways to lose weight, and there are better ways to prepare nutritious low-fat or no-fat snacks. They just don't make as much money for large companies.

PART III:
NOT ALL THE POISONS
WE DRINK ARE FOUND
UNDER THE SINK

DO YOU LIKE TO GET UP IN THE MORNING WITH YOUR FULLY LOADED COFFEE MAKER SET ON AUTOMATIC?

Sixteen

THIS IS YOUR HEART ON CAFFEINE . . .

D ID YOU REALLY like coffee the first time you drank it, or did you just acquire a taste for it? I drank coffee because of the way it made me feel, not because of the way it tasted. I thought it gave me a lot of energy. It allowed me to push myself past my normal state of endurance and continue to do things that I knew I probably shouldn't do— things like driving late, working late and studying late. I really enjoyed the extra activity that caffeine allowed me to accomplish. I didn't know it, but I was about to discover that not all the poisons we drink are under the sink.

There is a catch to this wonderful partnership that we forge with caffeine. When you rob from Peter to pay Paul, sooner or later you have to pay everything back—with interest. That is what happens when your adrenal system is constantly stimulated by caffeine. Sooner or later you are going to have to pay back your adrenal system and depleted energy reserves. When you try to pay back, you will discover that your body is charging you interest.

I promise you that your adrenal debt will have to be paid back sooner or later. While in graduate school at Florida State University, I was drinking as many as eighteen cups of coffee *each day!* When I was twenty-seven years old, I almost died of heart disease. The experience was very much like watching my life on a big screen, across which was written the headline, *This is your heart on caffeine!* The caffeine in the eighteen cups of coffee I was drinking every day wasn't the only reason this happened to me, but it was definitely one of the precipitating factors.

According to the British medical journal, *Lancet,* just five cups of coffee a day will increase a man's risk of heart disease by up to 50 percent. Women face a high risk in another area.

CAFFEINE IS AMERICA'S STIMULANT OF CHOICE

CAFFEINE, NUMBER EIGHT on our list of "Ten Foods You Should Never Eat," is the most widely used drug in our society. It can quickly stimulate the human brain, nervous system and adrenal glands, and it is very addictive and readily available. Caffeine shows up in everything from coffee, tea, chocolate and nearly every cola made on the planet to lesser-known sources such as aspirin products, analgesics and over-the-counter stimulants.

Dr. Reginald Cherry, author of *The Doctor and the Word,* makes a good point about coffee and caffeine that I feel I should pass along to you—even if it stops far short of my total abstention recommendation. In a chapter entitled "Foods That Fight Depression and Memory Loss," Dr. Cherry wrote:

> God has put it within man to seek out various things that can protect the mind and counter depression. Caffeine is a widely used mood elevator taken by millions of people. Studies show it can indeed function as a mild antidepressant through a complex effect on certain brain chemicals. Additional studies indicate caffeine can actually increase concentration, reaction times and thought processes. Don't exceed two cups of regular coffee daily. Certain people should avoid caffeine entirely (including those with irregular heartbeats or fibrocystic breast changes).[1]

Caffeine occurs naturally in coffee beans, tea leaves, cacao beans (chocolate), kolanuts (yes, there is such a thing) and other natural products. All of these products contain natural substances called *methylxanthines*—of which one is caffeine. When these substances occur naturally in plants, they act as pesticides against many kinds of insects. As with virtually any drug, caffeine has its positive attributes, but it has some very negative attributes—especially when it is abused or used excessively.

The pharmacological effects of caffeine include increased stimulation of the brain, the hormonal system, the excitory brain neurotransmitters and marked adrenal stimulation. When the adrenal glands are stimulated (as in the "flight-or-fight" response), glucose or blood sugar that is stored in the liver is released in mass quantities into the system. This is the "rush of energy" we feel when we are suddenly frightened, confronted with danger or receive a strong dose of caffeine.

CAFFEINE TAPS OUR EMERGENCY ENERGY RESERVE

THE TRUE PURPOSE of such strong adrenal response in our bodies is to provide emergency energy to our muscles so we can either fight for our lives or "fly" for our lives. Eventually—if this response is artificially invoked repeatedly through caffeine abuse or constant stress—this can lead to hypoglycemia, or low blood sugar and adrenal overload. Excess adrenaline in the body can be very detrimental if it is not burned up in a genuine "flight-or-fight" effort.

Caffeine can aggravate premenstrual syndrome in women.[2] It also increases stomach acid secretion, which can ultimately lead to heartburn or gastritis. This is why I recommend that everyone who is fasting or trying to reduce their weight phase out the coffee. Anyone who has ever ingested too much caffeine at night will also tell you that the drug will also promote sleeplessness and act as a diuretic (fluid loss from body tissues). This is no surprise, since "caffeine works by blocking one of the brain's natural sedatives, a chemical called *adenosine.*"[3] This symptom isn't hard to notice—it makes you thirsty and keeps you running to the bathroom at the same time. Caffeinated drinks can actually remove more water than is contained in the beverages themselves.

Pamela M. Smith, R.D., says that most caffeinated drinks, such as coffee, tea and most colas, "contain tannic acid, a product that interferes with iron and calcium absorption and competes for excretion with other bodily waste products such as uric acid…Men are particularly prone to uric-acid excesses. This is one reason why a glass of tea or coffee—although fluid based—just doesn't do the job."[4]

IMAGINE FIFTY CUPS OF COFFEE
IN YOUR SYSTEM!

A TYPICAL EIGHT-OUNCE cup of coffee contains between 50 and 150 milligrams of caffeine (instant coffee is the lowest; drip-brewed coffee is the highest). Decaffeinated coffee contains approximately 3 milligrams of caffeine. A cup of tea contains 50 milligrams of caffeine, while a twelve-ounce cola contains 35 milligrams. The average American consumes 150 to 225 milligrams of caffeine per day, with the vast majority of this coming from coffee consumption. Some people literally consume an excess of 7,500 milligrams of caffeine each day, or the equivalent of fifty cups of coffee!

Excessive consumption of caffeine—or caffeine abuse—can produce severe symptoms similar to those found in generalized anxiety and panic disorders. Extreme symptoms such as depression, nervousness, heart palpitations, general irritability, recurrent headaches and muscle twitching led psychiatrists, psychologists and other health professionals to coin the term *caffeinism* to describe this clinical syndrome. In fact, studies have shown that caffeine intake has been positively correlated with the degree of mental illness in psychiatric patients.[5]

Obviously, people with hypertension who are trying to keep their blood pressure under control should carefully avoid or stop drinking caffeinated beverages. Caffeine abuse is listed as one of the fifteen key risk factors for hypertension.[6]

I've already mentioned that the methylxanthine in caffeine increases a woman's risk of fibroid-tumor formation on breast tissue. It does this by stimulating growth of breast cells and causing painful enlargement of breast tissue and benign lumps, a condition known as *fibrocystic disease.*[7]

ELIMINATE THE OFFENDER

THE BEST WAY to deal with this condition once it is diagnosed is the least-followed procedure, even though it doesn't require minor surgery or biopsy, much less a radical procedure such as a mastectomy. Dr. John McDougall cites studies that indicate that in as many as *90 percent* of women with fibrocystic disease, these benign breast lumps significantly improve or completely disappear in two to six months when methylxanthines are eliminated from the diet.[8] There is also concern from investigators that the chronic stimulation of the breast tissue by methylxanthines may eventually progress to cancer of the breast in some women.[9]

In recent years, the public has become aware that caffeine has the potential of causing birth defects in unborn children. This is due partly to a fresh willingness on the part of physicians to tell their patients to avoid coffee, tea, colas and chocolate completely in all forms during pregnancy, which is in agreement with research findings on the subject.[10]

Dr. McDougall, in his book *The McDougall Plan,* notes that caffeine has been associated with cancer of the urinary bladder.[11] It has been associated with an increase in blood fats or triglycerides (*hypertriglyceridemia*), which itself may contribute to illness.[12] Caffeine may also cause the body to lose calcium.[13]

With these serious side effects in mind, my recommendation is that we wean ourselves off caffeine in all its forms—and then stay away from it! I promise you that you can live without it. I quit the caffeine habit. I have more energy now than I have ever had in my life, and I am in my forties.

I have a special concern for athletes who use caffeine as an athletic training tool. I got into the habit of drinking eighteen cups of coffee per day when I was an athlete at Florida State University.

A friend of mine used to say, "If I don't have a cup of coffee before I go to the gym, then I can't work out." He was overtraining, and he was exhausted because his body had been overstimulated with caffeine over an extended period of time.

THE PERPETUAL SEARCH FOR MUSCLE BURN

IF YOU ARE have been using caffeine as a stimulant while you train (power lifters and bodybuilders are some of the worst offenders because of their perpetual search for "muscle burn" and "the biggest lift"), then I urge you to be careful. The maximum limit of one or two cups of coffee that is recommended for optimum cardiovascular health will provide only a very short-term burst of energy. It usually takes very high levels of caffeine to produce a noticeable improvement in athletic performance. At the very least, those high levels of caffeine will leave you sleepless, anxious, jittery and blessed with an upset stomach and a headache.

In theory, large amounts of caffeine will create more energy by releasing free fatty acids in the liver, which can be used as an energy source, thus sparing the sugar (glycogen) stores in the muscles for later. However, caffeine is considered to be a drug and is banned by the International Olympic Committee (IOC), so not only do athletes run the risk of negative reactions to caffeine, but they may also risk losing the opportunity to compete. The IOC didn't order a total ban on caffeine since it is so common in beverages, but it did impose a maximum limit of 12 micrograms/milliliters of urine tested. An athlete would come very close to violating this limit if he or she ingested 800 milligrams worth of caffeine (five to six cups of strong coffee or a couple of espresso drinks) over a three-hour period.[14] (This fact was verified by Mary Lou Retton, Bonnie Blair and Carl Lewis when I was privileged to share the platform with them at a seminar and was personally able to ask them about caffeine being a banned substance in the Olympics.)

The problem is that the IOC's maximum legal limit for caffeine isn't high enough to allow the athletes to improve performance by saving the energy in their muscles. The only way to break into that "caffeine-driven hyperperformance mode" is to ingest so much caffeine that you nearly exceed the legal limit.

HEART ATTACK IN A CUP

IF YOU ARE an athlete, don't do it. It is a "heart attack in a cup" when combined with high-exertion trauma, and if you survive in the short term, you will inevitably face some kind of "payback" time when your adrenal system and your body demand compensation for your abuse. It won't be pretty.

Begin today to reduce the coffee, sugar and salt in your system. Replace these things with healthy alternatives like coffee substitutes—Postum, Caffix or Roma. Try some of the delicious herbal teas available instead. Just remember that caffeine is a robber. It will stimulate the system, but it will not provide *any* nutritive value.

When I was drinking eighteen cups of coffee a day, I knew that I was using the caffeine in the coffee as a stimulant—a "liquefied drug"—to increase my energy. I didn't realize at that time that caffeine causes your body's adrenal glands to over-work. In fact, I was to learn the hard way that overconsumption of caffeine over a long period of time could cause your body to go into adrenal exhaustion.

TOTALLY AND COMPLETELY ADDICTED

I WAS TOTALLY and completely *addicted* to caffeine. Are you? Do you like to get up in the morning with your fully loaded coffee maker set on auto-matic? I used to set my coffee maker to come on automatically about thirty minutes before I would get up because I loved to wake up to the smell of fresh perked coffee in the house.

It was my solemn ritual to sit there and get my charge of high-octane rocket fuel first thing in the morning just so I could get myself cranked up. I went so far as to tell my college roommates, "Look, don't talk to me. Don't come around me. Don't even breathe my air. Don't invade my space. In fact, don't have anything to do with me until I have had three or four cups of coffee."

When you are addicted to that much coffee per day—eighteen cups—everything seems to move in slow motion in the morning. You just wait, sometimes with cup in hand, for that percolator or drip coffee maker to finally crank up and deliver your morning dose.

Since I really didn't care for the *taste* of coffee, I used to fill my six-cup porcelain Swiss stein almost to the brim and immediately pour in whole milk for creamer, along with a sweetner. Then I would sit there and stare at the wall or watch television—just waiting for my "drug" to take effect so I would feel better.

The problem was that six cups of coffee was not enough. My health had deteriorated so badly by that time that as soon as I finished my first coffee stein of six cups and ate a high-protein meal for breakfast (which is what I should not have been eating), I would go back to bed. This went on for three months. (Remember, this is during the time I had been diagnosed with heart disease.)

Around lunch time I would start the "solemn ritual" all over again, only it was the "P.M. version." Basically I pulled myself out of bed again just to have another six cups of coffee. The process took place again that evening to round out my coffee and caffeine intake at a total of eighteen cups of coffee.

I STILL FIGHT THE CAFFEINE URGE

WHEN I EXPERIENCED my problems with my heart, I knew I had to find a way to wean myself off coffee. I was addicted to caffeine, but I did not accept it at the time. After years of drinking the stuff, I had convinced myself that I liked the taste of coffee. Every once in a while, I will *still* find myself thinking, *Well, maybe just a small cup of coffee... maybe just a little bit of coffee after dinner in this nice restaurant. I always have to fight these things to the finish because I know that if I allow myself to start drinking coffee again it would be very easy to once again become an addict.*

If you know that you are addicted to coffee, I do not want you to stop drinking coffee suddenly. That is not necessarily the healthiest way to do it. I consider it unhealthy to drop most addictions that quickly. In my case, I dropped from eighteen cups of coffee to seventeen cups on the first day. On the second day, I drank sixteen cups, then I dropped down to fifteen and fourteen and twelve and so on. Every day I would drop another cup of coffee until I finally got down to one cup of coffee a day. That is when the headaches started.

At first I literally thought I had a migraine headache because my head hurt so badly. Then I found that those headaches were a normal side effect of caffeine withdrawal. One time I felt so bad that I got up feeling nauseous and actually vomited. My head hurt, my eyes could not handle any light and I felt so emotionally fragile that I couldn't handle any pressure. I could not believe the intensity of the pain that was created by my withdrawal from caffeine.

After I cut my coffee quota to one cup, I hit a plateau of sorts. I didn't want to go any lower, but I knew I had to. My solution was to dilute one cup of coffee down to half a cup of coffee and half a cup of milk. Finally, I reached the point where I was drinking one-eighth of a cup of coffee and a half cup of milk! This went on for several weeks, after which I went ahead and went "cold turkey." Oh, the headaches...I couldn't believe it.

So That's Why I Feel So Bad

CAFFEINE CAUSES THE blood vessels in the brain to constrict. When you become addicted to caffeine, these blood vessels *stay* constricted on an ongoing basis. If for any reason you should not get your daily caffeine fix, these blood vessels dilate (or grow larger) and cause tremendous cranial pressure in your head, causing an incredible headache. Some of you are thinking, *That explains why I feel so bad when I don't get my coffee in the morning.*

I don't think we need to be addicted to any kind of drug to such a degree. Caffeine products stimulate the adrenals. When you overstimulate the adrenals, they go into exhaustion—a condition that is very unhealthy for your body.

After I managed to wean myself away from my coffee addiction, I was shocked at how exhausted I felt. But the improvement I saw in my health was incredible. I was still tired. The times I felt exhausted happened because I was still recovering from months and years of running on high octane at artificially sustained "fight-or-flight" emergency levels. My body was still purging itself of all the caffeine, sugar, high-fat dairy products and the five to ten Sudafeds I had taken on a daily basis for years and years. Can you believe that I had been pumping myself full of all those drugs *because I thought that was the way to stay healthy?* My philosophy was simple: I thought that it was effective to treat *symptoms* rather than *problems.* I had never been taught there was a difference.

I want to assure you that *there is life after caffeine.* I can look back on those days now and laugh about it. But I wasn't laughing back then—caught in the middle of a mess and flat on my back with my health collapsed. Many of the hundreds of thousands of people who hear me at seminars tell me that they are amazed at how quick and articulate my speaking is during my seminar presentation. I just have to laugh and tell them, "Listen, when I was in graduate school at Florida State University,

I used to drink a lot of coffee—eighteen cups a day. If you think I speak quickly *now,* you should have heard how quickly I spoke on eighteen cups a day!"

In summary, try to never drink coffee or other caffeine products. However, if you are going to drink coffee, at least do it in moderation. It is best if you avoid drinking coffee on an everyday basis, because this keeps the body from getting addicted to the artificial levels of stimulation provided by the caffeine. Once you make the break and endure the inevitable "separation anxiety" of weaning yourself from caffeine, you will feel better. That is a promise with which you can live.

TAKEN TOGETHER,
ALL THE STUDIES OF
WATER CHLORINATION
SUGGEST IT IS
STRONGLY ASSOCIATED
WITH CANCER,
ESPECIALLY IN THE
BLADDER AND RECTUM.

Seventeen

IT'S TIME TO COME CLEAN ABOUT CHLORINE AND FLUORIDE

THERE ARE TWO myths that have become fixtures in the minds of millions of Americans, due in part to skillful misinformation campaigns dating all the way back to the 1920s. It is time to come clean about the true story of chlorine and fluoride, two highly toxic poisons we routinely ingest while believing these substances "are there to protect us." We also need to avoid drinking them in our water supplies and scrubbing our teeth with them because together, they have earned a place on the "Ten Foods You Should Never Eat" list.

If you ever belonged to the Boy Scouts or the Girl Scouts as a kid, perhaps you remember being told that it is wise to carry along chlorine tablets in case your water runs low and you need to draw water from a stream. The idea was that you could drop a chlorine tablet in the water, and the water would be perfectly safe to drink as soon as the chemical had dissolved.

Veterans of the trench wars in France during World War I might have a different memory of chlorine. Before the "Great War," Germany was becoming very proficient at making dyes with derivatives of chlorine. When the war started and thousands of troops were hunkered down in trenches for months on end, the Germans came up with the idea of using highly toxic chlorine gas as a chemical weapon. They used to heat big vats of chlorine and remove the tops so the gas would blow downwind (or so they hoped) and kill the enemy troops. It was also during this time that chemical solvents were introduced.[1] During my college chemistry years, whenever we combined chemicals that had the potential to release chlorine gas, we always used a vaccum hood to pull the gas out of the lab—just one good inhalation of chlorine gas could send you to the hospital, or worse.

According to ecologist and biologist Sandra Steingraber, the waterworks of Boonton, New Jersey, became the first city to add chlorine to community water supplies. Chlorination was considered a cheap and effective way to stop epidemics carried by water during World War I. She writes, "By 1940, about 30 percent of community drinking water in the United States was chlorinated, and at present, about seven of every ten Americans drink chlorinated water."[2]

AVOID CHLORINE AND ITS
TRIHALOMETHANE OFFSPRING

THE PROBLEM WITH the popularity of water chlorination is twofold. First, chlorine gas is a dangerous poison in its own right, and over the last twenty years, the results of nearly two dozen studies "...have linked chlorination of drinking water to bladder and rectal cancers and, in some cases, to cancers of the kidney, stomach, brain and pancreas," according to Dr. Steingraber.[3]

Second, and possibly even more important, when chlorine reacts with organic contaminants such as dead leaves or other organic residues, it forms hundreds of different "organochlorine disinfection by-products." The EPA has found up to twelve hundred of these organochlorine volatiles in drinking water, some of which are carcinogenic. One of the most dangerous members of this family is a subgroup called *trihalomethanes*. Chloroform is one of the better-known members of this trihalomethane subgroup. Trihalomethanes are deadly because they can easily be ingested, inhaled and absorbed by our bodies.

According to Dr. Steingraber, all volatile organic compounds classified as trihalomethanes are regulated as a group (whenever they can be "contained"). She writes:

> Their maximum-contaminant level is 100 parts per billion. Their maximum-contaminant-level goal is zero. In the EPA's (Environmental Protection Agency) chart of drinking-water standards, along the row labeled "Total Trihalomethanes," is a single word: *cancer*.[4]

YOUR RISK GROWS THE MORE CHLORINATED WATER YOU DRINK

TAKEN TOGETHER, ALL of the studies of water chlorination suggest it is strongly associated with cancer, especially in the bladder and rectum. The association is strongest where above-ground sources such as rivers are the source of drinking water. Basically, the longer you drink chlorinated water (or shower in it or breathe the vapors while someone else does), the higher your cancer risk. (Dr. Steingraber has a personal interest in this issue because she was diagnosed with bladder cancer when she was still in her twenties. She lived to tell about it and to search out the causative agents behind the disease that tried to destroy her.)

We created many of our health problems ourselves through the misuse of chemicals and the contamination of natural resources. So many new degenerative conditions constantly arise that the medical profession is helpless to deal with them. All they can do is put labels on them. Many, if not most, of them stem from decades of contamination of the soil and water supplies with pesticides. We used these poisons indiscriminately for pest control because they attack the nervous systems of insects and rodents. Now they are attacking our bodies in much the same way, only they do it slowly in most cases. They collect in our bodies, particularly in our fat tissue, over long periods of time where they wait like time bombs. As soon as our immune-system threshold drops below the levels of toxicity in our bodies, disease manifests.

We put chlorine into our drinking water to kill live organisms, and this is often necessary. However, we should think seriously about getting the water as clean as possible before we add the chlorine to limit the production of lethal trihalomethanes. Then we could remove the chlorine before sending it out through the community water system to our children. The problem is that we forget that God designed us to be living organisms, too. Chlorine destroys our cells just as it destroys the cells of other living organisms.

MORE BAD NEWS ABOUT CHLORINE

IF YOUR WATER supply is chlorinated, have you noticed that your skin gets dry and your hair seems dry and frayed? That is part of the cosmetic package delivered by chlorine. We absorb chlorine through the skin, but we also drink that chlorine, and it destroys the intestinal flora or bacterial needed by the colon for proper digestion. Without this vital defense mechanism, the body is susceptible to a host of parasites and other disease organisms such as *Candida albicans* (yeast infections). If you recall our earlier discussions of how cholesterol can accumulate in the blood, then you should know that continual exposure to chlorine will also increase your risk of atherosclerotic plaquing because chlorine elevates LDL (bad) cholesterol.

Dr. Andleman, a key researcher at the University of Pittsburgh Graduate School of Health, conducted years of tests to see, in part, how water contaminants affect humans during the daily routines of bathing and showering. What he discovered can't be classified as good news.

We know that when we drink chlorinated water from the tap, we are often exposed to chlorine, trihalomethanes and other volatile organic chemicals. Unfortunately, Dr. Andleman discovered our exposure to these dangerous toxins was six to one hundred times *higher* in a hot shower or bath. It was the same if you even breathed the air around your dishwasher, washing machine or toilet! Why? Because these contaminants are airborne, and our bodies easily absorb them through the skin and the air we breathe. According to my friend and water purity specialist, Fred Van Lue, there are half a million households in this country that are literally drinking tap water that the EPA wouldn't even certify as safe for swimming![5]

ARE YOU SHARING A HOT TUB WITH CHLOROFORM?

CHLOROFORM WAS ONE of the first commercially popular trihalomethanes in this country. It became the anesthesia of choice for surgeons and dentists—until it was discovered that chloroform could cause cancer. Now it shows up mostly in the form of solvents, fumigants and as ingredients in refrigerants, pesticides and synthetic dyes. The human body can clear out this substance in about sixteen hours, but this isn't good enough. We are exposed to this carcinogen over and over again every day through the food we eat, the water we drink and the air we breathe. When you take a hot shower, you are breathing chloroform that is being released. Fred Van Lue says that when you are sitting in a hot tub, there is about one-thirtieth of an inch of pure chloroform sitting there with you. This trihalomethane is absolutely deadly to people who have heart problems. If you have heart problems, the last thing you should climb into is a heavily chlorinated hot tub.

Dr. Joseph Price told Fred Van Lue that chlorine poisoning contributes to many of the deaths of half a million people who suffer fatal heart attacks and strokes each year. He is personally convinced that in many of these cases, these incidents can be traced back to more than dietary problems—part of the blame must go to the high levels of chlorine in their water. He said this could be shown demographically because the areas of the country having the highest levels of chlorine in their public-water supplies also had the highest numbers of heart-disease patients. He said that there was a direct correlation between heart disease in Vietnam veterans and the heavy chlorination present in the water they were drinking while conducting jungle operations.[6]

Fred Van Lue has uncovered a lot of fraud and criminal activity tied in with the whole fluoride issue. He became personally involved after his son was poisoned with fluoride in 1987. That crisis propelled him full time into the water business. He told me:

I focused the same questioning attitude that I had used in my work in natural healthcare upon the water business. I had to. I had to find out how to avoid making the mistakes I made concerning the appropriate water treatment for my home. We had moved from an area in Massachusetts with a low dissolved-salt surface water that was chlorinated but not fluoridated. The system I chose failed to remove the fluoride from the heavily fluoridated high-dissolved salt water supply in the area of Texas where we settled down.

It wasn't long before my infant son began to have terrible reactions to the high fluoride levels in the water. The symptoms were horrible. He couldn't digest even his mother's milk once the fluoride took hold. He had perpetually sunken eyes, and his teeth came in months late. When they did come in, they looked as if someone had taken a shotgun to them, or as if they were made of Swiss cheese. He also had terribly stunted growth. It was just horrendous for my son and the whole family. Many months passed before we got it stabilized through a lot of natural healthcare, although even to this day you can still see some of the effects. My son is a great kid, and he's pulled out of it very well.[7]

ATHLETES ARE AT GREATER RISK

A SPECIAL POPULATION that is particularly at risk are athletes. Young athletes in high schools and colleges drink far more water and take showers more frequently than the general population because of their high exertion levels. We are beginning to see that they generally have more health problems in midlife. In fact, we are seeing young athletes in junior and senior high school beginning to drop dead of heart failure at alarming rates. Why? While the answer is probably complex, at least part of the equation should include the high volume of chlorinated water these athletes consume (an average of six to ten times more than the general population).

The more chlorine and fluoride you ingest, the more likely your risk of atherosclerotic plaquing and other forms of damage to the body. This gives us even more reasons to make sure our young athletes drink pure unchlorinated or dechlorinated water purified by reverse osmosis or steam distillation. In my experience, this argument has been a "hard sell" in junior high, high school and college athletic departments.

Dr. J. Peter Burts, of the EPA Toxicology Lab in Cincinnati, Ohio, was interested in doing research along the lines of previous work done by Dr. Joseph M. Price, whom we mentioned earlier. Dr.

Burts wrote to Dr. Price to say that he found that chlorine greatly depressed high density lipoprotein plasma in the body, and it increased the LDLs or low density lipoprotein plasma. This is significant because it is an established medical fact that HDL (the good cholesterol) helps prevent heart attacks. The chlorine we take in depresses HDL while it increases our levels of LDL cholesterol—which clogs the arteries.

Meet Chlorine's Twin Sister...

CHLORINE'S "EVIL TWIN sister" may be even more revered in the public's eyes than chlorine because most of us—and our children or grandchildren—meet this carcinogenic chemical up close as much as three times a day! I am referring to fluoride, which is produced in large scale as a by-product of aluminum.

Aluminum and fluoride are two of the most abundant substances found in the plant kingdom (in colloidal form), and neither of these substances are harmful to our bodies in this form. However, when your body comes into contact with the metallic form of aluminum, it goes berserk. Aluminum has the ability to pass right through the brain barrier just like lead, producing long-term but deadly results.

Frankly, fluoride acts like rat poison in your

body. If it doesn't kill you outright due to an over-dose, then it will begin to accumulate in your glands and fat tissues over time. The thyroid gland, the key administrator of your hormonal system, collects twice as much fluoride as any other organ in the body! Fluoride, however, is able to manifest itself in any organ. It is a total enzymatic poison that creates some of the rarest forms of cancers according to research conducted by the National Toxicology Group.

MORE TOXIC THAN LEAD

AFTER CONGRESS MANDATED the tests, the NTG found that some of the rarest sarcomas (cancers) in existence were caused by the ingestion of fluoride. If you look at a poison index, you will discover that fluoride is considered *more toxic than lead,* and only slightly less toxic than arsenic! (Do you still want to give it to your children?)

You probably didn't know that the metallic form of fluoride is a by-product of aluminum produc-tion. All you know is that from your childhood you have been told by responsible adults and an unending stream of TV commercials that fluoride is necessary for the prevention of tooth decay. Don't feel bad; you felt the way the fluoride inter-ests, toothpaste companies and advertising agencies wanted you to feel.

Evidently those organizations forgot to convince Merriam-Webster, the publisher of *Webster's Dictionary*. Fluoride can be present in many forms. One of the most common forms is sodium fluoride, which Webster's Dictionary describes as "a poisonous crystalline salt (NaF) that is used in trace amounts in the fluoridation of water, in metallurgy, as a flux and as a pesticide."[8] This same fluoride salt was, and still is, the active ingredient in many rodent poisons. That is comforting, isn't it?

The fluoride saga began during the era when the United States was dominated by a handful of powerful families in the late 1920s, including Andrew Mellon of the Mellon family. The Mellons owned Alco Aluminum, and they had a problem on their hands. The industry was having a serious problem with a waste by-product of aluminum production called *fluoride*. (This problem wasn't new in Europe. An aluminum smelter in Freiburg, Germany, in the mid-1800s, paid the first court damages on record to farmers because of the damage caused by the fluorides emitted from the smelter factory. A few years later, Italian aluminum manufactures were also forced to pay damages because of fluoride contamination around their smelters.)

TOXIC WASTE FOR SALE

EVEN BY THE turn of the century, fluoride problems were already turning up around Alco smelter sites in Colorado and in other areas as well. Andrew Mellon wanted to find a good (and profitable) use for fluoride so his company wouldn't be forced to dispose of it all as toxic waste. He needed to find a *big* use for it, because his plants were producing hundreds of thousands of tons of fluoride per year (they still are). Again, the metallic form of aluminum that is freed in the manufacturing process is very, very destructive to all life forms—plant, animal and human!

Then the Mellons heard about a small city in Texas that had *naturally occurring fluoride* in its water supply. This was attracting some attention because it was also noticed that its citizens had a lower incidence of dental cavities than that of people in other communities. It seems that the naturally occurring fluoride caused rapid collagen expansion, which caused the teeth of those Texans to harden and helped to prevent cavities.

Andrew Mellon moved quickly to set up a new government board called the Department of Natural Health (Mellon and other powerful financiers possessed much more power to influence government and government leaders in those days—as long as they were willing to pay for it).

Then Mellon installed the top lawyer at Alco Aluminum as the head of this new federal department. His first assignment was to set up a "Fluoridation Board" with but one task: *Find a good use for fluoride.*

The truth is that research does not support the decay prevention claims made for fluoride. As early as the 1940s, when fluoride was originally being pushed on our families by the Fluoridation Board, Mellon's researchers designed a study involving tests in two New York cities. Fluoride was added to the public drinking water system of Newburg, New York, while the water supply of the second city, Kingston, New York, was left untouched.[9]

YOU'LL GET CAVITIES AND CANCER, TOO

THE RESULTS WERE less than flattering. When the 4,969 school children of Newburg (the fluoridated city) underwent dental exams, 3,139 had tooth decay. Of the 5,308 children in fluoride-free Kingston, only 2,209 had tooth cavities.[10] Not only did fluoride fail to prevent dental decay, but in more recent years it has been shown to be carcinogenic!

In one study, forty-five to one hundred thirty-five parts per million (ppm) of sodium fluoride (NaF, the same formula found in toothpaste) caused changes in DNA synthesis in just four hours![11] What is more alarming is the fact that the dose of fluoride in toothpaste or mouthwash *is twenty-three times higher than those used in this experiment, suggesting a carcinogenic potential of these products as well.*[12]

Originally, the Fluoridation Board had envisioned a glowing ten-year comparative study. After four dismal years of watching the cavity curve go down instead of up in fluoride-free Kingston, the Fluoridation Board did what any respectable government entity would do when things go wrong: They quickly fluoridated fluoride-free Kingston (the city with superior dental records) and stopped the study. They weren't going to be bogged down by the facts.

THE STUDY YOU NEVER HEAR ABOUT

FLUORIDATION WAS PROMOTED across the country without a single study showing fluoride to be either safe or effective when taken internally. When the New York State Education Department conducted their own follow-up study with the same children in Newburg and Kingston, researchers found that there were *more* dental problems in the fluoridated city than in the fluoride-free city. Oddly enough, that study is never cited, even though its findings were personally presented before Congress by recognized scientific experts like Dr. John Yamitus, author of *Fluoride: The Aging Factor*, and the now deceased Dr. Dean Burk.[13]

The proof continues to surface time after time. When the city of Thurmond, Maryland, shut down its fluoridation pumps for repairs or maintenance, they noticed up to a 78 percent decrease of lead in their tap water. Why? Fluoride is so acidic that it severely corrodes lead pipes, lead pipe joint solders and almost any metal in general. It can eat through a one-inch iron pipe in a fluoridated water system in just a matter of months!

WHY ARE WE DOING THIS?

THE OFFICIALS IN Thurman never turned their fluoridation pumps back on. When they saw their lead levels drop 78 percent, it made them look at their fluoridation system and think, "Why are we even doing this?" The same thing happened in Tacoma, Washington. When they shut down their fluoridation pumps, they experienced a 50 percent decrease in tap water lead levels.

We are slowly learning that fluoride is a poisonous substance, despite all of the propaganda. Three people died in a Chicago teaching hospital in 1973 after their dialysis equipment failed to remove the fluoride in the drinking water before it was used during a dialysis procedure. The fluoride killed three patients and made several others extremely ill. This is the substance we are assured is so good and necessary for our children.

The truth is that a child has actually died of cardiac arrest in a dentist's chair while topical fluoride was being applied to his teeth. A $300,000-dollar award was paid to bereaved family members after a child made the mistake of swallowing the allegedly beneficial topical fluoride that the dentist put in the boy's mouth. Unfortunately, the dentist didn't know the child had swallowed the fluoride. When the boy got sick they couldn't catch it in time, and he died within a few hours. Fluoride is extremely poisonous, and it is a proven carcinogen.

HOW CAN WE REMOVE FLUORIDE FROM DRINKING WATER?

TWO METHODS WILL remove fluoride from municipally treated tap water. The first method is steam distillation, and the second method is reverse osmosis, which can easily be done at home using a variety of units available at reasonable prices. That is it. Carbon-block filters will not remove fluoride.

If your community fluoridates your water, don't drink it, and hardest of all, don't use fluoride toothpaste, fluoride drops or fluoride vitamins. It is a decision you can live with. We are the first generation that's having to suffer through the consequences of heavy fluoridation and heavy chlorination around the country. It is time for us to stop listening to the propaganda and start doing something to preserve our health and the health of our families.

ALCOHOL IS A
DRUG THAT HAS A
DEVASTATING EFFECT
ON NEARLY EVERY
MAJOR SYSTEM IN THE
HUMAN BODY—AND
IN HUMAN SOCIETY.

Eighteen

THE STAGGERING
TRUTH ABOUT
ALCOHOL PRODUCTS

ALCOHOL, THE FINAL member of the "Ten Foods You Should Never Eat" group, is a lethal substance inside our bodies. It kills brain cells, eats at stomach linings, erodes liver cells, inundates kidneys, attacks the pancreas, causes sclerosis of the liver, slows motor reaction times, grossly deforms unborn babies, contributes to osteoporosis, releases clouds of cancer-causing free radicals, weakens immune systems, robs the body of vital nutrients, raises blood sugar levels almost uncontrollably, causes alcoholism and helps trigger or worsen cancerous growths in the pancreas, liver, breast, bladder and esophagus. Alcohol is actually a drug that has a devastating effect on nearly every major system in the human body—and in human society.

Alcohol is even more deadly outside the body. It erodes the personality, removes protective inhibitions against dangerous behavior and fractures relationships with family members, spouses, friends and employers. It siphons off finances, shatters homes and makes orphans of innocent children. Alcohol kills thousands in drunk-driving tragedies every year. Alcohol is not a very nice drug.

Many Christians who attend my seminars bring up Paul's advice to Timothy in 1 Timothy 5:23: "Don't drink only water. You ought to drink a little wine for the sake of your stomach because you are sick so often." In this incident, Paul is concerned for Timothy who is having health problems—and dwelling at a location where water purity was questionable at best.

Even in that day, wine contained no contaminated water, only the juices extracted from grapes. Paul's advice was very wise and appropriate for his day and time. If Paul were writing to Timothy in modern America, he would probably advise him to avoid tap water in favor of purified water—and to avoid wine because of the tendency of the locals toward drunkenness and overindulgence in alcoholic products.

Was It Wine or Diet?

In 1977, a research study was released claiming that the residents of France had a lower incidence of heart disease than we do in this country because they drank red wine.[1] The truth of the matter is that the leading cause of death in France is *still* heart disease, but no one bothered to mention that fact. In addition to that, the French people have some of the highest incidences of pancreatic cancer, liver cancer, cirrhosis of the liver and alcoholism in the world.

I think their generally *superior diet* helped improve their national heart disease rates. Despite their taste for rich foods on occasion, the French as a whole tend to eat a much healthier blend of vegetables, fresh whole-grain breads and fruits than do Americans who love their fast foods. They don't use hydrogenated oils, and they use very little sugar. On the other hand, the *heavy wine consumption* of the French helped them win top honors in the alcohol-related disease categories.

We need to get a firm grip on reality. You don't need to drink red wine to reduce your risk of heart disease—take Vitamin E for heaven's sake! It is much more effective, and you won't have all the side effects associated with alcohol. We just don't need to use alcohol products in order to be healthy in this country. If alcohol could reduce the risk of heart disease, we would be one of the healthiest nations on earth! Instead, we are leading the world when it comes to heart disease, diabetes and cancer rates. I've never heard anyone say, "My life was a wreck, and then I started drinking and everything worked out OK." Isn't the opposite the truth for many alcoholics who started with just one social drink? Think about it.

Many cultures rely on locally made wines and beer as their primary beverage, some out of necessity, others for reasons of preference. My focus in this book is on this country, where wine, beer and hard liquor simply aren't necessary. We have our choice of hundreds of bottled and home-made beverages that do not contain alcohol. The physical, spiritual and social price tag on alcoholic beverages is simply too high. The proof is in the figures.

According to a study released in 1998 by the National Institute on Drug Abuse (NIDA), the National Institute on Alcohol Abuse and Alcoholism (NIAAA) and the National Institutes of Health (NIH), the economic cost of alcohol and drug abuse was estimated at *$246 billion* in 1992, the most recent year for which sufficient data was available.

This estimate represents $965 for every man, woman and child living in the United States in 1992. Alcohol abuse and alcoholism generated about 60 percent of the estimated costs ($148 billion), while drug abuse and dependence accounted for the remaining 40 percent ($98 billion).

Two-thirds of the costs of alcohol abuse related to lost productivity, either due to alcohol-related illness (45.7 percent) or premature death (21.2

percent). Most of this economic burden attributed to alcohol use falls on the shoulders of people who *do not abuse alcohol and drugs.* About 45 percent of the costs of alcohol abuse is borne by those who abuse alcohol and members of their households; 39 percent by federal, state and local governments; 10 percent by private insurance and 6 percent by victims of abusers.

We spend nearly four hundred billion dollars a year on alcohol products as a nation, but we pay a lot more for it in other ways. At least 107,400 deaths in 1992 were related to alcohol abuse. The NIDA report said, "Many of the alcohol- and drug-related deaths were among persons between ages twenty and forty, because the major causes of death, such as motor vehicle crashes [and] other causes of traumatic death...*are concentrated among younger-age cohorts.*" Alcohol abuse is estimated to have contributed to 25 to 30 percent of all violent crime.

AVOID ALCOHOL FOR THE CHILDREN'S SAKES

WE NEED TO understand how alcohol affects our youth. Such knowledge will be a strong motivating factor to convince us to stop using all alcoholic products—for our children's sakes if for no other! According to figures released by the Center for Substance Abuse Prevention:

- An alarming number of young people engage in harmful binge drinking (five or more drinks at one sitting): 15 percent of eighth graders, 25 percent of tenth graders and over 31 percent of twelfth graders.[2]

- Alcohol is a factor in the three leading causes of deaths among fourteen- to fifteen-year-olds: unintentional injuries, homicides and suicides.[3]

- Twenty-one percent of young drivers fifteen to twenty years of age who were killed in automobile crashes were intoxicated at the time of the incident.[4]

- Research suggests that alcohol use may lead to sexual aggression on college campuses. One study noted that 67 percent of male sexual aggressors and 50 percent of female victims had been drinking at the time the victimization occurred.[5]

- College students—many of whom are minors—who engage in binge drinking are seven to ten times more likely to have unplanned and unprotected sex, damage property, get into trouble with authorities or get injured.[6]

- Adolescent alcohol abusers show elevations in liver enzymes, an early indicator of liver damage.[7]

- Adolescent alcohol use is associated with earlier initiation of sexual activity, more frequent sexual activity and less frequent condom use.[8]

- The younger the age of drinking onset, the greater the chance that an individual at some point in life will develop a clinically defined alcohol disorder.[9]

THE HIGH COST OF PROMOTING DRUG USE

SOME OF AMERICA'S largest alcoholic beverage companies are putting their money into advertising directed to a target audience of young people. The CSAP report listed the following information:

- Expenditures for beer advertising totaled over $726 million in 1997. Television was the most widely used medium, with over $633 million spent on advertisements.[10]

- Since 1996 hard liquor has been advertised on TV and radio. Broadcast advertising spending nearly tripled between 1996 and 1997.[11]

- Mega-brewer Anheuser-Busch spent $1.3 million for each thirty-second commercial during the 1998 Super Bowl, and even more in 1999, despite the large number of kids who watch the game.[12]

The true cost of alcohol skyrockets when the choices we make ruin the lives of other innocent victims. This is never so true as with the unborn in what medical professionals call "fetal-alcohol syndrome." This refers to the risk that unborn children will endure the adverse effects of alcohol when their mothers drink while carrying them in the womb. These "adverse effects" range from growth deficiencies to brain structure and function anomalies and abnormalities of the head and face.[13]

Despite federally mandated warning labels on all alcoholic drinks and extensive public education campaigns, *four times* as many pregnant women frequently consumed alcohol in 1995 as in 1991, the year after the government began to require warning labels. One national survey found that more than half of all women ages fifteen to forty-four *drank while pregnant.*[14]

THERE IS A HIDDEN RISK TO ALCOHOL CONSUMPTION

IN ADDITION TO the highly visible costs and risks

associated with alcohol consumption, there is another more hidden but just as terrifying risk we take every time we decide to drink alcoholic beverages.

> Chemicals can cause other kinds of damage to tissues and vital organs, even though, as in cancer, the causative mechanism is not understood. In man, a prime example is alcohol, which used over a period of time can lead to cirrhosis of the liver—a hideous disease.[15]

Dr. Steingraber noted, "Drinking alcoholic beverages can cause a chemically induced, noncancerous growth to turn into liver cancer. In such a case, which kind of cancer is this: one caused by a lifestyle or by the environment?"[16]

Dr. John McDougall states in his book *The McDougall Plan:*

> Medical science has long been aware of the hazards associated with the use of alcohol, tobacco, caffeine and illegal drugs such as cocaine and marijuana...Several studies have demonstrated increased longevity and decreased risk of heart disease in people who consume alcohol moderately.[17] Those who consume alcohol may try to justify their

habit with these studies. However, alcohol cannot be generally recommended, primarily because so many people become addicted to this drug.

More than 7 percent of the adult population suffers from alcoholism, which results in decreased productivity, accidents, crime, mental and physical disease, and disruption of family life. Furthermore, any benefit of alcohol related to the risk of heart disease is offset by a rise in total deaths from other causes.[18]

Alcohol also provides seven "empty calories" per gram, which can lead to obesity. Other adverse effects of excess alcohol include high triglycerides (blood fat), liver disease, cancer, birth defects (fetal alcohol syndrome) and multiple vitamin deficiency diseases, such as scurvy from a lack of vitamin C, night blindness from a lack of vitamin A, pellagra from lack of niacin (B_3) and nervous system diseases such as Wernicke-Korsakoff Syndrome from deficiency of thiamin (B_1).[19]

Dean Ornish, M.D., weighs in on the alcohol debate with a strong right to the belly in this memorable excerpt from his book, *Eat More, Weigh Less:*

Why a Beer Belly Is Just That

Alcohol suppresses your body's ability to burn fat. When you drink alcohol, your body burns up fat much more slowly than usual. In one study, for example, researchers found that three ounces of alcohol reduced the body's ability to burn fat by about *one-third.*[20] So it is not just the calories and the fact that alcohol is converted into simple sugars that make it fattening, but also the way that alcohol throws off your body's normal disposal of fat in your diet.[21]

The Case of the Alcoholic Baboons

Dr. Kenneth H. Cooper has long led the way in the battle of the bulge and the struggle for higher levels of physical fitness in America. While studying the interaction of such things as alcohol and caffeine on antioxidants and other vitamins in the body, Dr. Cooper uncovered an unusual study that warns us that alcohol and good health—in this case, the vital antioxidant beta carotene—don't mix:

Toxic effects of beta carotene in normal, healthy people have not been reported unless the provitamin is taken *with relatively large amounts of alcohol or by heavy smokers.* This conclusion is based on a 1993 study at New York's Bronx Veterans Affairs Medical Center involving "alcoholic" baboons. The animals were given excessive amounts of alcohol plus 30 milligrams a day of beta carotene (the equivalent of 50,000 international units per day). The baboons taking alcohol and beta carotene suffered more severe liver damage than did another group taking only alcohol.[22]

My advice is to avoid the entire problem by avoiding alcohol. However, understanding human nature as I do, I want you to know that Dr. Cooper advises people who are taking the antioxidant beta carotene to limit their daily alcohol intake to the equivalent of no more than two average-sized four-ounce glasses of wine, or two beers, or one mixed drink. He emphasizes that *under no circumstances* should anyone take beta carotene if they drink heavily (four to six ounces of pure alcohol per day).[23]

If you like to straddle the fence and drink sparingly or moderately, then you should take beta carotene at least four hours before you ignore my advice and drink alcohol. In other words, take your beta carotene at breakfast.

THE TALE OF TWO THERMOGRAPHS

I WANT TO add another lethal habit to the list. It shares some of alcohol's extremely addictive and destructive characteristics, as well as its habit of targeting underage children with advertising campaigns; for that reason, we must *eliminate smoking.*

I taught a biology lab at Florida State University in 1977. We were teaching the students about thermographs, thermography, breast scans and mammography. We examined a thermographic study of blood oxygenation that spoke volumes about the hazards of smoking.

The researchers did a thermograph of a test subject's hand as a control or baseline point. A thermograph measures temperature and displays it as a color scale. Red or any other warm color in the red/yellow spectrum would imply a warmer image, which also indicates oxygen in the blood. The thermographic display of the subject's hand was totally red, indicating that fully oxygenated blood was circulating through it.

Then the test subject—a smoker—was asked to inhale cigarette smoke *one time* and wait thirty seconds (no, he didn't have to hold his breath that long). When the subject's hand was placed back into the thermograph, his entire hand had turned blue! A single inhalation of cigarette smoke had robbed an extremity like the hand of almost all its oxygen source in the blood.

Let me end by returning to the beginning: Alcohol is one of the "Ten Foods You Should Never Eat," and for good reason. You have just waded through more statistics on alcohol and alcohol abuse than you ever wanted to see, and I applaud you for it. Now for the bottom line: Are you really determined to get *maximum energy* so you can live life to the fullest and fulfill your destiny? Even if that means you have to give up alcoholic beverages? As always, the decision is yours. It has nothing to do with whether or not you "go to heaven," but it may help determine "how quickly you get there." Whatever you do, make a decision with which you can live.

YOUR HEALTH IS
YOUR MOST VALUABLE
EARTHLY ASSET; WHAT
YOU DO WITH IT IS
YOUR RESPONSIBILITY.

Conclusion

ACHIEVE MAXIMUM HEALTH AND ENERGY ONE CHOICE AT A TIME

M Y DESIRE IS to see people walk in good health and prosper in everything they attempt. The apostle John summed up the way I feel when he prayed, "Dear friend, I am praying that all is well with you and that your body is as healthy as I know your soul is" (3 John 2).

Since I believe very strongly that God orchestrates certain "divine appointments" in our lives, I have to believe that it was no accident that this book landed in your hands. Perhaps you made the decision to pull it from a book shelf in a bookstore or to borrow it from a friend, but we know who is behind it, "for God is working in you, giving you the desire to obey him and the power to do what pleases him" (Phil. 2:13).

After a quarter of a century of studying human health and nutrition and its relationship to God's

Word, I have developed some strong convictions that are clearly expressed in the chapters you've read. Experience has revealed the sad reality that no matter what I do, some of the people reading these words won't be here in two years—they will die prematurely as I nearly did. It will happen because they didn't realize what the choices they were making in food and lifestyle were doing to the biochemistry of their bodies.

My goal has been to equip you with knowledge about your body and to remind you that your Creator intended for you to live life "more abundantly"—in maximum energy and health in this life. Your body is a tool to perform your will, and *you* are a tool in God's hands to perform His will. Computer programmers coined a phrase several decades ago that fits our discussion perfectly. The acronym for the phrase was G-I-G-O. It stands for "Garbage In; Garbage Out." I couldn't say it better, and ironically, this phrase is very biblical. It applies to every part of our being: body, soul and spirit.

LIVE ONE CHOICE AT A TIME

AS A BIOCHEMIST and nutritionist, I've come to understand this truth in ways I never knew existed thirty years ago. We must live our lives *one choice at a time,* knowing that every good choice we make will help build the foundation for a good life tomorrow and for a decade from now.

I was still in high school when I finally decided that I had had enough. It was time for a change. By God's grace, I took *personal responsibility* for my health and dietary choices. I was tired of looking and feeling the way I did, so I began to change my opinions and attitudes about dietary choices and exercise. I was in the tenth grade before it dawned on me that I could look better and feel better than I did. I have continued making choices that improve my health to this day—and will as long as I live. Really, it doesn't matter whether you are ten or one hundred years old. If you change your mind and attitudes today, you can improve the way you look and feel within thirty days. It all begins with a choice with which you can live.

I remember a thirty-three-year-old man who came into my office with a blood pressure reading of 180/120. He knew it was time for a change in his life, so he went on our Eat, Drink and Be Healthy program to change his lifestyle and eating habits. Thirty days later, he returned to his cardiologist and learned that his blood pressure had dropped to 120/70 without any drugs, liquid diets, fasting, appetite suppressers or quack food diets.

He started to avoid bad foods while eating good foods (all he wanted). He began exercising moderately on a consistent basis and supplementing his meals with key vitamins, antioxidants, minerals and trace minerals. In other words, he began to apply the same principles you read about in this book. That was years ago, but today his blood pressure is still perfect. His new life began with one decision and the courage to act upon it.

NOW WHAT?

YOU HAVE PLOWED your way through eighteen chapters of material covering elements of basic biochemistry, chemical contamination, molecular theories of the cell and free radicals, digestive processes, antioxidants and their interaction with precancerous and cancerous cells and, of course, the "Ten Foods You Should Never Eat." At this point you are probably thinking, *Now what?!*

I have done the only thing that I can do. I've armed you with information, and I've done everything I know to motivate you and help you to make choices for a lifetime. Many of the things we've examined together have been contrary to everything you and I were taught as kids (and as adults for that matter). I am sure some of it was absolutely aggravating. If I pressed too hard at times, I did it with the best of motives. (Many times emotion will precipitate change.)

Perhaps you picked up this book because your doctor just told you that your blood tryglicerides and cholesterol levels are alarmingly high. Or, you may have read this book just hoping that *this time,* you will find a way to take off the excess weight and keep it off. There is an outside chance that you were tempted to bypass all of the discussions about fat and cholesterol—you were after the *maximum energy* we promised on the front cover. So be it.

Now it is up to you to convert the knowledge you've gained into proven wisdom. In one sense, the difference between knowledge and wisdom is the *repeated application* of that knowledge. If you are at the point where I was back in the tenth grade, then you are sick of the high blood pressure, the fluctuating blood sugar levels and the pounds that keep creeping back no matter how many diets you start (and break). You have reached a plateau in your personal exercise regimen, and no matter what you do, you can't seem to advance any further.

Do you associate so much pain with the obstacle before you that you *are willing to do whatever it takes?* Good. Are you ready to make the decisions and commitments it will take to change your lifestyle? I'm asking this question because you will need *commitment* if you really want to press through the difficulty of change so you can feel good and look good for the rest of your life.

Be Reasonable

Attitude is very important, and you need to set specific (but reasonable) health and fitness goals to stay motivated. Nearly all of us are overweight, and the first and most logic goal for most people is to trim down to their ideal weight. (Be reasonable—if you are six feet tall with large bones, you know you should weigh more than one hundred pounds.) Don't set some lofty or unreasonable goal by saying, "I'm going to lose one hundred fifty-five pounds this year." You may very well lose a lot of weight when you begin to eat right and exercise regularly—*but you will do it one pound at a time.*

In the beginning, the aim is to get you to work out long enough to *develop a habit.* For some people, it only takes two to three weeks to make regular exercise and healthier food choices into a satisfying habit. For most of us, it will take three to six weeks to undo years of little exercise and poor eating habits. This is where step by step, *measurable goals* come in. They constitute small rewards for a job well done, along with a reminder that the difficulty of the first three to six weeks will produce more energy, self-assurance and good health for the rest of your life. Trust me on this: If you refuse to give up, if you continue to work out until it becomes a healthy habit, then you have successfully launched a new lifestyle with an invaluable energy advantage.

AIM FOR SOMETHING GOOD THAT IS WORTH THE EFFORT

YOU WILL BE a lot happier and more focused when you have something to shoot for. If you are shooting for the sky and you hit the wall, at least you hit *something*. If you don't plan for success, then you will get that for which you planned—nothing. Keep your eyes on the big picture. You are out to establish a new lifestyle, not to follow every caloric guideline.

I can promise you that you may slip from time to time. The most important thing I can tell you is this: *Never skip meals or go on a "diet"* (unless you fast for religious reasons). It is better to eat a little less but eat more often than to skip meals. This keeps your body metabolism higher so it won't go into a starvation mode and begin to hoard energy in the form of body fat.

TAKE ACTIONS *NOW*

IT IS IMPORTANT to take action *now*. Do what you have to do to achieve good health and maximum energy. The worst thing you can do is to read this book from cover to cover and then just sit around saying, "*Some day* I am going to lose this extra weight," or "*Some day* I am going to stop eating this junk food and start exercising so I'll look and feel better." If you want it bad enough, you will stop talking and take action now. If you need additional help, please call my office and order my Eat, Drink and Be Healthy program along with a delicious recipe guide. You can reach us at (800) 726-1834.

DO WHATEVER YOU DO CONSISTENTLY

MOST AMERICANS FALL into one of two categories when it comes to dietary changes or exercise. They closely match one or the other of the classic characters in the parable of the tortoise and the hare. If you recall this story from your childhood years, the tortoise was slow, plodding and consistent. The hare was extremely fast, but he was easily distracted, bored and lacked the ability to see a thing through. When the two competed against one another in a race, the tortoise ultimately won the race *because he was consistent.* Don't try to achieve your weight-loss goals or exercise goals in a single burst of extreme exertion or abstinence from food. Consistency will carry the day.

Consistency is the absolutely critical ingredient to success in every area of life. It makes the difference in our service to God, in our relationships with spouses and children and in our work. It is especially important in our journey to maximum energy and optimum health.

Conclusion

We have discussed a number of important keys to maximizing your energy. Do you remember them?

Keys to Maximize Your Energy

- Set a goal to do more than merely sustain life. Choose nutritious foods that will maintain health and provide you with the maximum levels of energy.

- Drink at least eight glasses of *pure water* per day. Drink even more water when you begin your new exercise program. Water is essential for good health and maximum energy.

- Make sure your diet includes adequate amounts of natural fiber—it is crucial if you really want to enjoy maximum energy and good health.

- Supplement your daily meals with vitamin and mineral supplements. Take extra care to get the antioxidants your body needs to help ward off cancer and other destructive diseases.

- Make sure you get your daily requirements of essential fatty acids—the Omega-3 and

Omega-6 oils are crucial to your body's health and proper metabolism. This is most easily done with supplements of flaxseed oil, evening primrose oil and cod liver oil in convenient capsule form.

- Exercise correctly and *consistently.* This is the secret to increasing your basal metabolic rate—the rate at which your body burns calories. It also helps to protect you from heart disease and various blood sugar level disorders.

- Learn how to manage stress effectively and to properly maintain your body's fundamental needs. It is the only body you have, so take care of it so it will serve you well.

THE TEN FOODS YOU SHOULD NEVER EAT

WE ALSO EXAMINED the "Ten Foods You Should Never Eat" list. Are they still burned into your memory? How about the specific items that are your personal favorites? Look at this summary so they will be fresh in your mind, and remember that each of these foods made the list for some very scientific reasons. They are biochemical outlaws that rob your body of needed nutrients, antioxidants and health levels. Seriously consider removing them permanently from your dinner table and refrigerator.

1. Avoid high-fat luncheon meat and all pork products—especially bacon, sausage, hot dogs and pepperoni (formerly my favorite carcinogen carrier). They will provide nothing for your body except extreme amounts of saturated fat, sodium, artificial food coloring and, worst of all, sodium nitrites. These ingredients actively convert to cancer-causing nitrosamines in your intestinal tract. Avoid them at all costs.

2. Remove shellfish from your personal menu. These scavengers from the sea are either carrion-eaters (such as lobsters, the giant cockroach of the sea) or filter-feeders. They all frequent the bottom of our planet's lakes, rivers and oceans. They are literally the "cesspools of the sea." What they collect, you collect when you eat them. This includes a vast array of parasites, environmental contaminants, viruses and bacterial agents that can be lethal.

3. Avoid the heart-stopping charms of margarine products—including partially hydrogenated vegetable oils such as Crisco shortening, most commercial brands of peanut butter and margarine. None of it is good for you.

4. Avoid the bitter bite of aspartame. This "artificial sweetener" known to most people as NutraSweet is actually a chemical that will wreak havoc inside your body and foster the development of a whole host of unpleasant diseases and health problems. Even white sugar is better than aspartame.

5. Leave the junk food behind. These sugary, high-fat items provide "empty calories" at best, and they are treated with a long list of preservatives so they will stay "fresh" on grocery shelves for months (or decades). Try reading the entire list of ingredients of one of these prepackaged items before you buy it— you probably won't want it after you've waded through that unpronounceable and indigestible list. These preservatives will do the opposite to your health. Choose healthy vegetable and fruit

snacks instead. You will live longer and feel better.

6. Avoid the "new fake fat" called olestra or Olean. It's chief strength is that it is the only fake fat that is able to escape the heat of a frying pan. All the others break down under high heat. Unfortunately, this stuff *never breaks down*. It just slides through the system untouched by stomach acids and enzymes—but it has a deadly tendency to take all of the essential fat-soluable nutrients and vitamins in your food along with it!

7. Avoid the twin sisters of the tap-water world: chlorine and fluoride. Both of these chemicals are classified as toxic poisons, yet our municipal water departments around the nation insist on polluting community water systems with dangerous levels of these chemicals. Do what it takes to provide pure, uncontaminated water to yourself and your family.

8. Wean yourself from high-fat dairy products. This group of foods may well be the primary culprits behind the fattening of America. High-fat cheeses are

particularly dangerous offenders because they show up on our pizzas, in our casserole dishes and on most of the hamburgers eaten in this country. They will help clog up your arteries faster than almost anything else.

9. Imagine your heart on caffeine—overworked, never allowed to reach its true resting state and ready to break down in heart-stopping fatigue. Caffeine is a drug that is extremely addictive and dangerous to your cardiovascular health (this is why doctors warn patients with hypertension to avoid coffee). Slowly wean yourself away from coffee, tea, colas and chocolate. Your heart and nervous system will appreciate it—once the headaches stop.

10. Recognize the staggering truth about alcohol, America's favorite drug of choice. It is highly addictive and highly destructive to our bodies, our families and our society. We are better off without it.

Do yourself a favor. Make your decision to pursue good health with an *energy advantage* today.

Then set practical and measurable step-by-step goals with which you can live. Finally, major on the majors and minor on the minors. Require yourself to make reasonable progress in a reasonable time. Don't expect perfection or rigid adherence to rules and guidelines.

You are out to build a healthier lifestyle, which is nothing more than "a consistent pattern of good choices made one at a time." This alone will take a lot of stress out of your life and release extra energy so you can pursue activities that really matter. With that said, let me end as I began.

Your health is your most valuable earthly asset; what you do with it is your responsibility. My prayer for you echoes the words of the apostle John written almost two thousand years ago:

> Dear friend, I am praying that all is well with you and that your body is as healthy as I know your soul is.
>
> —3 JOHN 2

NOTES

CHAPTER ONE
DISCOVERING THE KEYS TO GOOD HEALTH

1. "Dietary Goals for the United States," Washington, D.C.: Government Printing Office, stock no. 052-070-03913-2; cited by John A. McDougall, M.D., and Mary A. McDougall, *The McDougall Plan* (Piscataway, NJ: New Century Publishers, 1983), 13–14.
2. McDougall, *The McDougall Plan,* 6.

CHAPTER TWO
SUPPORT LIFE OR SUSTAIN HEALTH?

1. This is a statement by Dr. Richard Brannon, chairman of the board of trustees for the International Academy of Preventive Medicine.
2. Harvey Diamond, *Fit for Life* (New York: Warner Books, 1985).
3. There are many physical and spiritual benefits to fasting, but most of the physical benefits are limited to the shorter fasts. Anyone contemplating an extended fast of ten days or more should consult with a knowledgeable health provider, and would be wise to "work up" to the longer fast by conducting shorter, safer fasts first. This is a very important and somewhat complex subject that deserves detailed treatment. I have taught extensively on this subject, and I welcome you to contact our office for more information about available audio cassette tapes and material.

CHAPTER THREE
PURE WATER: THE GREATEST OF ALL "HEALTH POTIONS"

1. Cited by Mr. Fred Van Lue in seminar presentations.
2. Ibid.
3. Fred Van Lue developed a device being used by many cutting-edge golf courses called an "ESP," or essential energy system. It is an electrostatic precipitator that purifies water and places an ionic charge on it, which allows it to penetrate soils more efficiently and bond with fertilizers. It can be absorbed by grasses and trees more rapidly. The ESP system greatly reduces the amount of water needed to effectively produce results in agricultural applications. It also reduces the amount of chemical fertilizers or pesticides required *by up to 95 percent* while producing far superior results.
4. Cited by Fred Van Lue in seminar presentations.
5. Excerpt from a taped interview with Fred Van Lue, founder, WaterWise, Inc., in the tape entitled, "Water: Why You Absorb As

Many Toxins in One Hot Shower As If You Had Drunk 8 Glasses of Contaminated Water," Tape 8 of my tape series Forever Fit at 20, 30, 40 & Beyond.

CHAPTER FOUR
NATURAL FIBER—CRUCIAL TO HEALTH AND ENERGY

1. V. E. Iron interview, *Healthview Newsletter,* Issue 1, 1983.

2. J. F. Franklin and M. I. Chatton, *Current Medical Diagnosis and Treatment* (Los Altos, CA: Lang Medical Publishing, 1984).

3. D. Y. Graham, et al, "The Effect of Bran on Bowel Function in Constipation," *American Journal of Gastroenterogy,* 77, 599–603, 1982.

4. H. Andersson et al, "Transit Time in Constipated Geriatric Patients During Treatment With a Bulk Laxative and Bran: A Comparison," *Scandinavian Journal of Gastroenterology,* 14:821–826, 1979.

5. H. Trowell, D. Burkitt and K. Heaton, *Dietary Fibre, Fibre-Depleted Foods and Disease* (London: Academic Press, 1985).

6. Joseph E. Pizzorno, N.D., and Michael T. Murray, N.D., *Encyclopedia of Natural Medicine* (Seattle, WA: Bastyr College Publications, 1993).

7. D. S. Gray, "The Clinical Uses of Dietary Fiber," *American Family Physician,* 5(92):419–26, February, 1995.

8. D. J. Webster, D. C. Gough, and J. L. Craven, "The Use of Bulk Evacuation in Patients With Hemorrhoids," *British Journal of Surgery,* 65:291–2, 1978. Also see F. Mosesgaard, M. L. Nielsen, J. B. Hansen and J. T. Knudsen, "High-Fiber Diet Reduces Bleeding and Pain in Patients With Hemorrhoids," *Dis Colon Rectum,* 25:454–6, 1982.

9. M. M. Baig, J. J. Cerda, "Pectin: Its Interaction With Serum Lipoproteins," *American Journal of Clinical Nutrition,* 34:50–53, 1981.

10. L. A. Simons, et al, "Long-term Treatment of Hypercholesterolemia With a New Palatable Formulation of Guar Gum," *Atherosclerosis,* 45(1):101–108, 1982.

11. R. E. Hugh, "Hypothesis: A New Look at Dietary Fiber," *Human Nutrition: Clinical Nutrition,* 40C:81–86, 1986.

12. See the American Cancer Society, *Cancer,* 34(2):121–6, 1984; B. Reddy, "Metabolic Epidemiology of Large Bowel Cancer," *Cancer,* 42:28–32, 1978; and M. Hill, "Colon Cancer: A Disease of Fiber Depletion or Dietary Excess," *Digestion,* 11:289, 1974.

13. P. Greenwood, E. Lanza, "Dietary Fiber and Colon Cancer," *Contemporary Nutrition,* 11(1):1986.

14. B. J. Howie, T. D. Schultz, *American Journal of Clinical Nutrition,* 423:127–34, 1985.

15. M. S. Rosman, "The Effect of Long-Term High-Fibre Diets in Diabetic Patients," *South African Medical Journal,* 63(9):310–13, 1983.

16. See H. Philipson, "Dietary Fibre in the Diabetic Diet," *Acta Med Scan* (supplement) 671:91–93, 1983; and T. Poynard, et al, "Reduction of Post-Prandial Insulin Needs by Pectin As Assessed by the Artificial Pancreas in Insulin-Dependant Diabetics," *Diabetes & Metabolism,* 8(3):187–89, 1982.

17. M. L. Burr, et al, "Dietary Fibre, Blood Pressure and Plasma Cholesterol," *Nutritional Research,* 5:465–72, 1985.

18. J. Anderson, "Plant Fiber and Blood Pressure," *Annals of Internal Medicine,* 98:842, 1983.

19. See J. Kelsay, "Effect of Fiber From Fruits and Vegetables on Metabolic Responses of Human Subjects," *American Journal of Clinical Nutrition,* 31:1149, 1978; A. J. Silman, "Dietary Fibre and Blood Pressure," *British Medical Journal,* Jan. 26, 1980, 250; and A. Wright, et al, "Dietary Fibre and Blood Pressure," *British Medical Journal,* 2:1541, 1979.

CHAPTER FIVE
SUPPLEMENT YOUR DIET WITH VITAMINS
(ESPECIALLY THOSE VITAL ANTIOXIDANTS)

1. McDougall, *The McDougall Plan,* 7.

2. "Position of The American Dietetic Association: Vitamin and Mineral Supplementation," www.eatright.org/asupple

3. Source unavailable.

4. Kenneth H. Cooper, M.D., *The Antioxidant Revolution* (Nashville, TN: Thomas Nelson Publishers, 1994), 184.

5. Ibid., 8–9.

6. Ibid., 185.

7. Ibid., 190–191.

8. Dean Ornish, M.D., *Eat More, Weigh Less* (New York: HarperCollins Publishers, Inc., 1993), 30.

9. Source unavailable.

10. D. A. Wagner, et al, *Cancer Research,* 45:6519–22, 1985.

11. W. R. Bruce, P. W. Dion, "Studies Relating to a Fecal Mutagen," *American Journal of Clinical Nutrition,* 33:2511, 1980.

12. K. N. Prasad, et al, "Vitamin E Increases the Growth of Inhibitory and Differentiating Effects of Tumor Therapeutic Agents on Neuroblastoma and Glioma Cells in Culture," Proc Soc Exp Biol Med, 164(2): 158–63, 1980.

13. Wagner, *Cancer Research.*

14. H. B. Stahelin, et al, *Journal of the National Cancer Institute,* 73:1463–8, 1984.

15. R. B. Shekelle, et al, "Dietary Vitamin A and Risk of Cancer in the Western Electric Study," *Lancet,* November 28, 1981, pp. 1185–90.

16. J. S. Orr, et al, *American Journal of Obstetrics and Gynecology,* 151:632–5, 1985; and C. La Vecchia, et al, "Dietary Vitamin A and Risk of Invasive Cervical Cancer," *International Journal of Cancer,* Vol. 34:319–22, 1984.

17. G. F. Combs, L. C. Clark, "Can Dietary Selenium Modify Cancer Risk?" *Nutrition Review,* 43:325–31, 1985.

18. "Serum Vitamin and Provitamin A Levels and the Risk of Cancer, *Nutrition Review,* 42(6):214–5, 1984.

19. See J. Salonen, et al, "Risk of Cancer in Relation to Serum Concentrations of Selenium and Vitamin A and E: Matched Case-Control Analysis of Prospective Data," *British Medical Journal,* 290:417, 1985; G. N. Schrauzer, et al, "Cancer Mortality Correlation Studies—III: Statistical Associations With Dietary Selenium Intakes," *Bioinorganic Chemistry,* 7:23, 1977; and K. P. McConnel, et al, "The Relationship Between Dietary Supplementation and Breast Cancer," *Journal of Surgical Oncology,* 15(1):67–70, 1980.

20. I recommend 1 to 2 ounces of a high-quality colloidal trace mineral supplement such as AquaTrace every day. This will supply you with all of the minerals, trace minerals, rare-earth elements and organic compounds your body needs each day.

CHAPTER SIX
TAKE YOUR DAILY DOSE OF ESSENTIAL FAT!

1. McDougall, *The McDougall Plan,* 204.

2. Pamela M. Smith, R.D., *Eat Well, Live Well* (Lake Mary, FL: Creation House, 1992), 19.

3. Abstracts: The Netherlands Society for the Study of Diabetes, *Netherlands Journal of Medicine,* 29(2):65–70, 1986.

4. A. Houtsmuller, et al, "Favorable Influences of Linoleic Acid on the Progression of Diabetic Micro- and Macroangiopathy," *Nutrition Metabolism,* 24(Supp. 1): 105–118, 1980.

5. McDougall, *The McDougal Plan,* adapted from information provided on pages 14–15.

6. Ornish, *Eat More, Weigh Less,* 20.

7. Ibid., 22.

CHAPTER SEVEN
CHOOSE EXERCISE—IT'S A DECISION YOU CAN LIVE WITH

1. David J. A. Jenkins, et al, "Glycemic Index of Foods: A Physiological Basis for Carbohydrate Exchange," *The American Journal of Clinical Nutrition,* Vol. 34, March 1981, 362–366.

2. Contact my office at (941) 967-8284 for more information about the Glycemic Index and how it can be used to make wise food choices.

3. We have developed a comprehensive, three-level exercise program and video that covers the do's and don'ts of exercise in great detail. It is tailored to meet the different needs of beginners, regulars and full-time or professional athletes. Call my office for more information at (800) 726-1834.

CHAPTER NINE
AVOID THE CONCEALED DANGERS IN
HIGH-FAT LUNCHEON MEAT

1. I am not saying that these treatments should never be used. There are some natural alternative treatments that cancer patients might want to consider before they commit to more invasive and destructive treatments. In most cases, there is enough time to try the conventional treatments should alternative treatments fail to be effective. In all cases, I urge patients to consult closely with their primary healthcare provider, preferably a physician who is willing to consider carefully the patient's concerns and wishes.

2. The National Academy of Sciences, *Nutrition, Diet, and Cancer,* 1982.

3. Professor Hans-Heinrich Reckeweg, M.D., "The Adverse Influence of Pork Consumption on Health," *Biological Therapy,* Volume One, Number Two, 1983.

4. United Nations Department of International Economic and Social Affairs, "Comparison of Infant Mortality Rates in Industrialized Countries," a table showing the infant mortality rates among twenty industrialized nations for babies who die before one year of age. Figures were compiled from the last available figures supplied by the respective nations for the years 1985, 1986 or 1987.

5. Ralph W. Moss, Ph.D., "Link Between Trophoblasts and Cancer Corroborated," cites a landmark article published in mid-1995 by Hernan F. Acevedo, Ph.D., et al, of the Allegheny-Singer Research Institute, Pittsburgh, in *Cancer*, 1995; 76: 1467–1475. Dr. Moss writes, "Acevedo is well-known for his prior work confirming some of the assertions of *Virginia Livingston-Wheeler*, another doctor whose treatment was enriched by the Beardian thesis. Using conventional and accepted methods, this time Acevedo rigorously showed that the 'synthesis and expression of hCG...is a common biochemical denominator of cancer.'" Dr. Moss is the author of eight books and three documentaries on cancer-related topics. He is an advisor on alternative cancer treatments to the National Institutes of Health,

Columbia University, and the University of Texas. He researches and writes individualized "Healing Choices" reports for people with cancer.

CHAPTER TEN
SIDESTEP THE HIDDEN HAZARDS OF SHELLFISH

1. Sandra Steingraber, Ph.D., *Living Downstream: A Scientist's Personal Investigation of Cancer and the Environment* (New York: Vintage Books, a Division of Random House, Inc., 1997), 132–134.
2. Ornish, *Eat More, Weigh Less*, 34–35.
3. News Release issued in 1999 by Mike Ostasz, Division of Environmental Health, Alaska Department of Environmental Conservation, 555 Cordova Street, Anchorage, AK 99501-2617.
4. Steingraber, *Living Downstream*, 142.
5. Ibid.
6. Ibid., 140.
7. Quoted from an official CDC warning notice posted on the U.S. Government's official CDC web site at http://www.cdc.gov/ncidod/diseases/foodborn/ vibriovu.htm

CHAPTER ELEVEN
LEAVE YOUR "JUNK" BEHIND

1. Sharon's *Eat, Drink and Be Healthy Cookbook* is a phenomenal cookbook featuring the healthy foods and cooking methods prominently mentioned in this book. You may contact Broer & Associates at (800) 726-1834 for more information.
2. See G. Fara, "Epidemic of Breast Enlargement in Italian School," *Lancet*, 2:295, 1979; and C. Saenz de Rodriguez, "Environmental Hormone Contamination in Puerto Rico," *New England Medical Journal*, 310:1741, 1984.

CHAPTER TWELVE
WEAN YOURSELF FROM HIGH-FAT DAIRY PRODUCTS

1. Ornish, *Eat More, Weigh Less*, 34.
2. McDougall, *The McDougall Plan*, 5.
3. See McDougal, *The McDougal Plan*, 5; as well as J. Bayless, "Lactose and Milk Intolerance: Clinical Implications," *New England Journal of Medicine*, 292 (1975):1156; "Background Information on Lactose and Milk Intolerance," *Nutrition Reviews*, 30(1972):175; and T. Gilat, "Lactase Deficiency: The World Pattern Today," *Israel Journal of Medical Science*, 15(1979):369.
4. J. Gordon, "Weanling Diarrhea," *American Journal of Medical Science*, 245(1963):129.

5. Robert S. Mendelsohn, M.D., *How to Raise a Healthy Child... in Spite of Your Doctor* (New York: Ballantine Books, 1984), pg. 52.

6. S. Bahna, *Allergies to Milk* (New York: Grune and Stratton, 1980).

7. Adapted from McDougall, pg. 52, who cites three original sources: R. Fontaine, "Epidemic Salmonellosis from Cheddar Cheese: Surveillance and Prevention," *American Journal of Epidemiology,* 111(1980):247; K. Donham, "Epidemiologic Relationships of the Bovine Population and Human Leukemia in Iowa," *American Journal of Epidemiology,* 112(1980):80; and J. Ferrer, "Milk of Dairy Cows Frequently Contains a Leukemongenic Virus," *Science,* 213(1981):1014.

8. See McDougall, page 50, citing E. Eastman, "Adverse Effects of Milk Formula Ingestion on the Gastrointestinal Tract—An Update," *Gastroenterology,* 76(1979):365; and A. Cunningham, "Lymphomas and Animal Protein Consumption," *Lancet,* 2(1976):1184.

9. Steingraber, *Living Downstream,* 9–10.

10. McDougall, page 145, citing A. Strom, "Mortality From Circulatory Diseases in Norway 1940–1945," *Lancet,* 1(1951):126; and page 45, citing J. Stamler, "Lifestyles, Major Risk Factors, Proof and Public Policy," *Circulation,* 58(1978):3.

CHAPTER THIRTEEN
THE HEART-STOPPING TRUTH ABOUT MARGARINE PRODUCTS

1. H. B. Fu, et al, "Dietary Fat Intake and the Risk of Coronary Heart Disease in Women" (abstract), *New England Journal of Medicine,* 1997 Nov. 20;337(21): 1491–1499.

2. M. W. Gillman, et al, "Margarine Intake and Subsequent Coronary Heart Disease in Men," *Epidemiology,* 1997 Mar; 8(2):144–149.

3. L. Kohlmeier, et al, "Adipose Tissue Trans Fatty Acids and Breast Cancer in the European Community Multicenter Study on Antioxidants, Myocardial Infarction, and Breast Cancer," *Cancer Epidemiology, Biomarkers & Prevention,* 1997 Sep; 6(9):705–710.

4. Udo Erasmus, *Fats That Heal, Fats That Kill* (Burnaby, BC, Canada: Alive Books, 1993), 103.

5. For more information on the FDA, along with voluminous documentation, read *Eating May Be Hazardous to Your Health: How Your Government Fails to Protect You From the Dangers in Your Food,* by Jacqueline Verrett, Ph.D., and Jean Carper (New York: Simon and Schuster, 1974).

CHAPTER FOURTEEN
THE BITTER FACTS ABOUT ASPARTAME AND DIET SODAS

1. L. Stegink, L. J. Filer, Jr., "Aspartame," Marcel Dekker, Inc. (1989).

2. G. D. Searle Company, Confidential internal memorandum titled,

"Food and Drug Administration and other Drug Sweetener Strategy." Documents supplied by Senator Howard Metzenbaum's office (December 28, 1970).

3. *Steadman's Medical Dictionary*, 25th edition (Baltimore, MD: William and William, 1990).

4. R. J. Louis, *Sax's Dangerous Properties of Industrial Materials*, Eighth Edition (New York: Van Nostrand Reimhold, 1992), 2251–2252.

5. Ibid.

6. W. Monte, "Aspartame: Methanol and Public Health." J Appl Nutr 36:42–54, 1984.

7. See D. Thomas-Dobersen, "Calculation of Aspartame Intake in Children," *Journal of the American Dietetic Association*, 89(6): 831–833 (1989); and Federal Register 44:31716–31718 (June 1, 1979).

8. Federal Register 38:5921 (March 5, 1973).

9. Federal Register 39:27317 (July 25, 1985).

10. See Federal Register 46:38285 (July 24, 1981) and U.S. Court of Appeals for the District of Columbia Circuit, No. 84–1153. Community Nutrition Institute, et al., Petitioners v. Dr. Mark Novitch. Acting Commissioner, Food and Drug Administration, Respondent. G. D. Searle Co., Inventor, Petition for Review of an Order of the Food and Drug Administration. No. 84–5253 Community Nutrition Institute, et al., Appellants v. Dr. Mark Novitch, Acting Commissioner, Food and Drug Administration, Appellee (September 24, 1985).

11. See documents supplied by Senator Howard Metzenbaum's office in February 6, 1986, and Federal Register 40:56907 (December 5, 1975).

12. Food and Drug Administration Searle Investigation Task Force chaired by Carlton Sharp. "Final Report of Investigation Review of G. D. Searle Company" (March 24, 1976).

13. Federal Register 44:31716–31718 (June 1, 1979).

14. H. J. Roberts, "New Perspectives Concerning Alzheimer's Disease," *On Call*, August 1989.

15. Letter from Richard A. Merrill, Chief Counsel, Department of Health, Education and Welfare, Food and Drug Administration, to Honorable Samuel K. Skinner, U.S. Attorney, Northern District of Illinois, requesting that Skinner's office convene a Grand Jury investigation into G. D. Searle Co. for submitting false reports, dated January 10, 1977.

16. Letter from Howard J. Trienens, Sidley & Austin, to Samuel K. Skinner, U.S. Attorney, Northern District of Illinois (January 26, 1977).

17. Documents supplied by Senator Howard Metzenbaum's office (February 6, 1986).

18. Confidential memorandum from Samuel K. Skinner, U.S. Attorney, Northern District of Illinois, to William Conlon and Fred Branding. Document supplied by Senator Howard Metzenbaum's office. (March 8, 1977).

19. Memorandum from Charles P. Kocoras, First Assistant U.S. Attorney, to Samuel J. Skinner, U.S. Attorney, regarding the G. D. Searle Company (April 13, 1977).

20. Documents supplied by Senator Howard Metzenbaum's office (February 6, 1986).

21. Food and Drug Administration, J. Bressler, "The Bressler Report, investigation of Searle Laboratories" (August 7, 1977).

22. See Memorandum from Bureau of Foods Task Force, Food and Drug Administration, to Howard R. Roberts, Ph.D., Acting Director, Bureau of Foods, regarding "Authentication Review of Data in Reports Submitted to the Food and Drug Administration Concerning Aspartame" (September 28, 1977); U.S. General Accounting Office's "Briefing Report to the Honorable Howard Metzenbaum, U.S. Senate: Food and Drug Administration. Six Former HHS Employees' Involvement in Aspartame's Approval" GAO/HRD-86-109BR (July 1986); documents supplied by Senator Howard Metzenbaum's office (February 6, 1986); and U.S. General Accounting Office's "Report to the Honorable Howard M. Metzenbaum, U.S. Senate: Food and Drug Administration. Food Additive Approval Process Followed for Aspartame," GAO/HRD-87-46, Common Cause (June 1987).

23. Federal Register 44:31716–31718 (June 1, 1979).

24. See Food and Drug Administration Public Board of Inquiry, W. J. H. Nauta, P. W. Lampert, V. R. Young, "Aspartame" (Docket No. 75F-0355): Decision of the Public Board of Inquiry" (September 30, 1980); Federal Register 48: 54993–54995 (December 8, 1983) and Federal Register 46: 38288–38289 (July 24, 1981); and U.S. Court of Appeals for the District of Columbia Circuit, No. 84-1153.

25. See Committee on Labor and Human Resources, "NutraSweet—Health and Safety Concerns, Hearing Before the Committee on Labor and Human Resources, U.S. Senate, One Hundredth Congress, First Session on Examining the Health and Safety Concerns of NutraSweet (Aspartame)" (November 3, 1987); and Federal Register 46:50947 (October 16, 1981).

26. See U.S. Court of Appeals for the District of Columbia Circuit, No. 84-1153; and Federal Register 47:46140 (October 15, 1982).

27. Food and Drug Administration, "Aspartame in Carbonated Beverages Approved," FDA Talk Paper (July 1, 1983).

28. Federal Register 48: 31376 (July 8, 1983).

29. Congressional Record 131(58): S5489–S5517 (May 7, 1985).

30. F. Graves, "Results of *Common Cause* Magazine Investigation of FDA's Approval of Aspartame," *Common Cause* (July 1984).

31. Centers for Disease Control, Division of Nutrition, Center for Health Promotion and Education, "Evaluation of Consumer Complaints Related to Aspartame Use" (November 1984).

32. Ibid.

33. J. Zaslow, "Searle's John Robson to Remain in Two Posts Until After Merger," *Wall Street Journal* (October 1, 1985).

34. G. R. Verrilli, A. M. Muser, *While Waiting: A Prenatal Guidebook,* (St. Martin's Press, 1986).

35. Documents supplied by Senator Howard Metzenbaum's office (February 6, 1986).

36. Letter from John M. Taylor, Associate Commissioner for Regulatory Affairs, Food and Drug Administration, to James S. Turner, Swankin & Turner, denying the Community Nutrition Institute's petition to seek administrative reconsideration of GDA's regulations concerning Aspartame (November 21, 1985).

37. Committee on Labor and Human Resources (November 3, 1987).

38. Letter from John M. Taylor (November 21, 1986).

39. Letter from F. Owen Fields, Ph.D., Novel Ingredients Branch, Division of Product Policy, Center for Food Safety and Applied Nutrition, Department of Health and Human Services regarding "Pre-1988 Aspartame Approvals" (February 25, 1994).

40. U.S. General Accounting Office, "Report to the Honorable Howard M. Metzenbaum, U.S. Senate: Food and Drug Administration, 'Food Additive Approval Process Followed for Aspartame,'" GAO/HRD-87-46, Common Cause (June 1987).

41. Department of Health and Human Services, Health and Injury-Related Surveillance Subprogram Postmarketing Surveillance System, "Quarterly Report on Adverse Reactions Associated with Aspartame Ingestion," submitted to Health Hazards Evaluation Board (January 2, 1987).

42. NutraSweet Company, "U.S. Consumer Products Containing NutraSweet Brand Sweetener" (February 2, 1988).

43. See Food and Drug Administration Department of Health and Human Services, "Quarterly Report on Adverse Reactions Associated with Aspartame Ingestion" (October 1, 1988); and Department of Health and Human Services, "Report on All Adverse Reactions in the Adverse Reaction Monitoring System" (February 25 and 28, 1992).

44. W. Monte, "Aspartame: Methanol and Public Health," J Appl Nutr 36:42–54, 1984.

45. Ibid.

46. R. G. Walton, "Seizure and Mania After High Intake of Aspartame," *Psychosomatics* (March 1986).

47. H. J. Roberts, "Aspartame (NutraSweet): Is It Safe?" The Charles Press (1990).
48. Mary Nash Stoddard, Aspartame Consumer Safety Network, P.O. Box 780634, Dallas, TX 75378, (214) 352-4268.
49. C. Gaffney, Armed Forces Institute of Pathology, "Aspartame in Aviation." Paper presented at the 57th Annual Scientific Meeting of the Aerospace Medical Association (April 1986).

CHAPTER FIFTEEN
HOLD THE OLESTRA AND LIVE LONGER

1. "Summary: Olestra in the Gastrointestinal Tract," published by Proctor & Gamble, 1998.
2. Ibid.
3. Ibid.
4. "CSPI protests deceptive labeling and advertising. Warns of health risks from fake fat," Center for Science in the Public Interest (CSPI) New Release, June 10. Internet: http://www.cspinet.org
5. "Fake-fat Olestra Sickens Thousands, 15,000 Cases Makes Olestra Most-Complained-About Additive Ever," Center for Science in the Public Interest (CSPI) New Release, Dec. 22, 1998. See http://www.cspinet.org for more information.
6. "CSPI protests deceptive labeling and advertising. Warns of health risks from fake fat," Center for Science in the Public Interest (CSPI) New Release, June 10. Internet: http://www.cspinet.org
7. "Olestra 'Snack Attack' Hits Thousands of Hoosiers: Victims Go on Protest March to State Health Department," Center for Science in the Public Interest (CSPI) New Release, July 15, 1997. Internet: http://www.cspinet.org
8. *Advertising Age,* June, 1998, published by Crain Communications, Inc.
9. "CSPI protests deceptive labeling and advertising. Warns of health risks from fake fat," Center for Science in the Public Interest (CSPI) New Release, June 10. Internet: http://www.cspinet.org
10. Ibid.
11. Ibid.
12. "Olestra 'Snack Attack' Hits Thousands of Hoosiers: Victims Go on Protest March to State Health Department," Center for Science in the Public Interest (CSPI) New Release, July 15, 1997. Internet: http://www.cspinet.org
13. "CSPI protests deceptive labeling and advertising. Warns of health risks from fake fat," Center for Science in the Public Interest (CSPI) New Release, June 10. Internet: http://www.cspinet.org
14. *Medical Sciences Bulletin,* published by Pharmaceutical Information Associates, Ltd., January 1996;18(5):3.

15. "FDA Approves Fat Substitute, Olestra," Pharmaceutical and Biotechnology Press Releases, Jan. 24, 1996.
16. "The Problems With Olestra," Center for Science in the Public Interest (CSPI), nd. Internet: http://www.cspinet.org
17. *American Journal of Clinical Nutrition*, 62:591 (1995).
18. *Journal of Nutrition*, 119:123-6 (1989); *American Journal of Clinical Nutrition*, 53(1 Suppl):238#-246S (1991).
19. *American Journal of Epidemiology*, 135: 115 (1992).
20. "The Problems With Olestra," Center for Science in the Public Interest (CSPI), nd. Internet: http://www.cspinet.org
21. Ibid.
22. Ibid.
23. "P&G, Frito-Lay, Set to Unleash Diarrhea-causing Olestra on Americans," Center for Science in the Public Interest (CSPI), News Release, Feb. 5, 1998. Internet: http://www.cspinet.org

CHAPTER SIXTEEN
THIS IS YOUR HEART ON CAFFEINE

1. Reginald Cherry, M.D., *The Doctor and the Word* (Lake Mary, FL: Creation House, 1996), 130.
2. Pamela M. Smith, R.D., *Food for Life* (Lake Mary, FL: Creation House, 1994), 88.
3. Ibid.
4. Ibid., 85.
5. See A. Neims and R. von Borstel, "Caffeine: Metabolism and Biochemical Mechanisms of Actions," in *Nutrition and the Brain*, Vol. 3, R. Wurtman and J. Wurtman, eds (New York: Raven Press, 1983); D. Charney, G. Henninger and P. Jotlow, "Increased Anxiogenic Effects of Caffenin In Panic Disorders," *Archives of General Psychiatry*, 41:233–43, 1984; J. Greden, P. Fontaine, M. Lubetsky and K. Chamberlin, "Anxiety and Depression Associated With Caffenism Among Psychiatric Patients," *American Journal of Psychiatry*, 131:1089–94, 1979; and S. Bolton and G. Null, "Caffeine, Psychological Effects, Use and Abuse," *Journal of Orthomolecular Psychiatry*, 10:202–11, 1981.
6. Norman E. Kaplan, *Clinical Hypertension* (Baltimore, MD: Williams and Wilkins Publishing, 1990).
7. J. Milton, "Response of Fibrocystic Disease to Caffeine Withdrawal and Correlation of Cyclic Nucleotides with Breast Disease," *American Journal of Obstetrics and Gynecology*, 135 (1979):157.
8. See P. Brooks, "Measuring the Effect of Caffeine Restriction on Fibrocystic Breast Disease," *Journal of Rep Med*, 26(1981):279; and J. Milton,"Response of Fibrocystic Disease to Caffeine Withdrawal…"

9. J. Elliot, "Cyclic Nucleotides as Predictors of Benign to Malignant Progression of Breast Cancer," *Journal of Rep Med,* 26 (1981): 279.
10. McDougall, *The McDougall Plan,* 175.
11. See P. Cole, "Coffee Drinking and Cancer of the Lower Urinary Tract," *Lancet,* 2(1971): 1335; and L. Marrett, "Coffee Drinking and Bladder Cancer in Connecticut," *American Journal of Epidimiology,* 117(1983): 113.
12. J. Little, "Coffee and Serum-Lipids in Coronary Heart Disease," *Lancet,* 1(1966):732.
13. P. Brooks, "Measuring the Effect of Caffeine Restriction...," 279.
14. "Caffeine and Athletic Performance," John Hopkins University Health Information Center, InteliHealth Internet Site, last updated August 14, 1998.

CHAPTER SEVENTEEN
IT'S TIME TO COME CLEAN ABOUT CHLORINE AND FLUORIDE

1. Steingraber, *Living Downstream,* 96–97.
2. Ibid., 202.
3. Ibid.
4. Ibid., 203.
5. Excerpt from a taped interview with Fred Van Lue, founder, WaterWise Inc., in the tape entitled, "Water: Why You Absorb As Many Toxins in One Hot Shower As If You Had Drunk 8 Glasses of Contaminated Water," Tape 8 of my tape series, Forever Fit at 20, 30, 40 & Beyond.
6. Ibid.
7. Van Lue interview.
8. *Webster's Ninth New Collegiate Dictionary* (Springfield, MA: Merriam-Webster Inc., 1988), 1120.
9. Morris A. Beale, *The New Drug Story* (Washington, D.C.: Columbia Publishing Co., 1958), 127.
10. Ibid.
11. T. Tsutsui, et al, "Induction of Unscheduled DNA Synthesis in cultured human oral keratinocytes by sodium fluoride," *Mutation Research,* 140:43–48, 1984.
12. PRN Sutton, "Letter to the editor," *New Zealand Medical Journal,* 98(775):207, 1985.
13. *Fluoride: The Aging Factor,* by Dr. John Yomitus, is an excellent book that is filled with easily understood charts and graphs, and a clear description of all the different tests that have been done showing that fluoride is a carcinogenic free-radical. If you read this phenomenal book, you will never put fluoride into your system again.

Chapter Eighteen
The Staggering Truth About Alcohol Products

1. K. Yano, "Coffee, Alcohol, and Risk of Coronary Heart Disease Among Japanese Men Living In Hawaii," New England Journal of Medicine, 297(1977):405.

2. L. D. Johnston, P. M. O'Malley, and J. G. Bachman, (1998). National Survey Results on Drug Use from the Monitoring the Future Study, 1975–1997. Volume 1: Secondary School Students (p. 126). Rockville, MD: U.S. Department of Health and Human Services.

3. U.S. Department of Health and Human Services. Healthy People 2000: National Health Promotion and Disease Prevention Objectives. (1991). NIH Publication Number (PHS) 91-50212. Washington, DC:U.S. Government Printing Office.

4. National Highway Traffic Safety Administration. (1998). Young Drivers Traffic Safety Facts 1997. Web Publication (URL: http://www.nhtsa.dot.gov/ people/ncsa/Young97.html).

5. M. P. Frinter and L. Rubinson, (1993). "Acquaintance Rape: The Influence of Alcohol, Fraternity Membership, and Sports Team Membership," Journal of Sex Education and Therapy, 19(4):272–284.

6. H. Wechsler, A. Davenport, G. Dowdall, B. Moeykens, and S. Castillo (1994). "Health and Behavioral Consequences of Binge Drinking in College: A National Survey of Students at 140 Campuses," Journal of the American Medical Association, 272(21):1672–1677.

7. A. M. Arria, M. A. Dohey, A. C. Mezzich, O. G. Bukstein, and D. H. Van Thiel (1995). "Self-Reported Health Problems and Physical Symptomatology in Adolescent Alcohol Abusers," Journal of Adolescent Health, 16(3):226–231.

8. M. L. Cooper, R. S. Peirce, and R. F. Huselid (1994). "Substance Use and Sexual Risk Taking Among Black Adolescents and White Adolescents," Health Psychology, 13(3):251–262.

9. National Institute on Alcohol and Alcoholism, (January 14, 1998), "Age of Drinking Onset Predicts Future Alcohol Abuse and Dependence," NIH News Release.

10. Beer Handbook (New York: Adams Business Media, 1998).

11. Liquor Handbook (New York: Adams Business Media, 1998).

12. G. Johnson, "Advertisers and Markets Are in the Lineup for $uper Bowl Sunday," Los Angeles Times, Business and Technology Section, January 8, 1998.

13. E. Abel, and R. Sokol, "Incidence of Alcohol Syndrome and Economic Impact of FAS-related Anomalies," Drug and Alcohol Dependence (1987), 19:51–70.

14. U.S. Department of Health and Human Services, *Substance Abuse and Mental Health Statistics Source Book,* 1998 (Rockville, MD: Substance Abuse and Mental Health Services Administration, 1998).
15. Verrett, *Eating May Be Hazardous to Your Health,* 68.
16. Steingraber, *Living Downstream,* 96–97.
17. Dr. McDougall includes this statement in his book, originally cited in Yano, "Coffee, Alcohol and Risk of Coronary Heart Disease Among Japanese Men Living in Hawaii," from the *New England Journal of Medicine.*
18. This paragraph cited in McDougall's quote was originally cited in W. Blackwelder, "Alcohol and Mortality: The Honolulu Heart Study," *American Journal of Medicine,* 68(1980):164.
19. McDougall, *The McDougall Plan,* 174–175.
20. This statement was originally cited in P. M. Suter, Y. Schutz, and E. Jequier, "The Effect of Ethanol on Fat Storage in Healthy Subjects," *New England Journal of Medicine,* 1992, 326(15):983–7.
21. Ornish, *Eat More, Weigh Less,* 39.
22. Cooper, *Antioxidant Revolution,* 121–122. This original study, included in Dr. Cooper's book, was originally cited in "Alcohol and Beta Carotene: A Cocktail Lethal to the Liver," *Environmental Nutrition,* February 1993, 8.
23. Cooper, *Antioxidant Revolution,* 122.